The Practice of Yoga brings us face to face with the extraordinary complexity of our own being.

— Sri Aurobindo of Auroville

Watch your thoughts; they become words. Watch your words; they become actions. Watch your actions; they become habits. Watch your habits; they become character. Watch your character; for it becomes your destiny.

— Upanishads

Yoga cultivates the ways of maintaining a balanced attitude in day to day life and endows skill in the performance of one's action.

— B.K.S. Iyengar

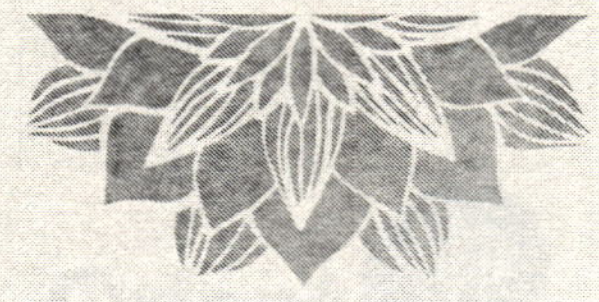

My heartfelt gratitude to Swami Kuvalayananda, Founder-Director of the Scientific Institute for Yoga Research, Lonavla, who has guided me and provided immense help throughout my research on Yoga therapy.

www.orientpaperbacks.com

ISBN : 978-81-222-0583-1

The Complete Book of Yoga: Harmony of Body and Mind

Subject: Health & Fitness / Yoga

Ist Published 1981
2nd Revised Edition 2017
Reprinted 2019
Reprinted 2026

Published by
Orient Paperbacks
(A division of Vision Books Pvt. Ltd.)
5A/8, Ansari Road, New Delhi-110 002

Asanas photographs by Anjali Devi Anand, teacher of Hatha Yoga at the Centre Indien de Yoga, Paris, and Sri Ananda

Cover design by Vision Studio

Printed and bound at
Saurabh Printers, Noida

Foreword

There is an immutable interchange and reciprocal dependence between body and soul. To affirm the body is to affirm the unity hidden behind the body-soul-mind complex. The body cannot on its own assert an existence that is separate from this unity. Any discipline that prepares the body to assume its role as the effective element promoting this unity may one day become the way towards the realisation of the Self. Seen in this light, Hatha-Yoga, which is first and foremost a method designed to turn the body into the perfect instrument, may be called the way to Self-realisation (Self being the body-mind-soul complex). The body is a sign, a language of God and of the Supreme. How can this 'sign' be improved so that we may communicate better with God and enlarge our understanding of what He tells us?

The interchange between body and soul is made clear by Prana, a neutral principle that is neither solely physical nor uniquely spiritual.

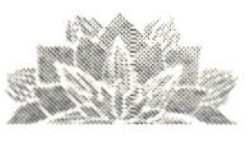

Hatha-Yoga attaches great importance to Prana and to breathing through alternate nostrils according to a certain rhythm; the same is true of the breathing that accompanies postures. The fact that we are able to relax the body is due to the thought (or conscience) that lies behind it. If someone says to me 'Relax', my first reaction is to tense up, and only afterwards relax. Why is this? The answer is that the body at first reacts unsuccessfully to the order; then thought, feeding the body, carries out the order and is able to make the body relax. The messenger that interprets and puts into action the order of the thought is Prana or Pranic energy. In the case of illness for example, Prana is the conductor-wire directing our will to recovery.

The present work is doubly important. Firstly, because the author, Sri Ananda, learnt Hatha-Yoga in a highly traditional way from a guru. Hence he is both careful and wise to stress the importance of breathing — a cardinal element of Hatha-Yoga. Secondly, he has lived in Europe and has come to understand their needs, bringing them a technique of unquestionable authenticity. It is striking to see how the declarations made by ancient Indian contemplative thinkers on the human body have been confirmed by science. The Yogis stated the sacred nature of the spine, in the centre of which is the Sushumna, the field of all great spiritual exprience. Hatha-Yoga advocates several postures to exercise the spine.

Science has confirmed by the experimental method what the Yogis discovered through meditation and intuition. The contemplative thinkers in India have a great contribution to make to the active non-contemplative West, but by accepting the practice of Hatha-Yoga and other methods of yoga, the West shows itself both receptive and spiritually open. Hence a living bridge has been created between the East and the West. The present work is eminently suited to its aim of enabling everyone to attain the harmony of body and mind, thus helping to make that bridge even stronger.

— Swami Nityabodhananda
Ramakrishna Mission, India

Introduction

Yoga is a science as well as a method that allows man to live a harmonious life while favouring his spiritual progress through the control of mind and body. The Asanas (Yogic postures) and Pranayama (breath control), better known as Hatha-Yoga, are a practice which not only help one acquire perfect health, stay young and live longer, but is designed to develop the inner force that enables us to overcome our failings and withstand stressful situations with serenity. It prepares the body for higher stages of yogic practice — such as concentration and meditation. Hatha-Yoga thus complements Raja-Yoga, whose supreme goal is the attainment of the state of Super-consciousness.

The great yogis tell us that those who know how to combine yogic postures (Asanas), breathing exercises (Pranayama), and the control of the mind or concentration (Dharana) may attain a state of perfection. The object of the Asanas and Pranayamas is the improvement of the physical body, while the control of the mind, i.e., the constructive power of the consciousness, is beneficial to the inner force, developing a positive, optimistic outlook on life; it

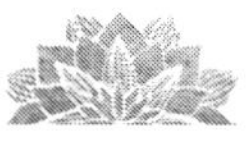

eliminates the fear of premature old-age and death, bringing with it a state of serenity. In my own experience and that of my pupils, the practice of the Asanas and Pranayama has undoubtedly shown the value of this discipline. I am convinced that a frail body is not only vulnerable and prone to illness, but also presents an obstacle to the development of mental forces and the improvement of self-expression. A balanced, healthy body is an important prerequisite for clear thought and a step on the way to concentration. I also believe that a person who is harmoniously balanced, both physically and mentally, can reach a very high level in terms of his consciousness and inner force, as well as developing his mental and spiritual forces to the utmost.

The object of Yoga is to enable us to reach a better knowledge of ourselves. It lays the foundations for a higher level of self-development and a deeper self-awareness. Above all, Yoga teaches us self-discipline, for very little can be achieved without it. Sometimes, however, discipline thus acquired can become extremely unbending and one-sided, leading to fanaticism and preventing future progress. Hence, the true way of obtaining the desired results lies in a self-discipline that is balanced.

Yoga is not a religion; it is the search for the inner development of the consciousness, going directly to the very heart of reality. It does not involve blindly obeying traditional rules; it is a way of progressively realizing one's full potential, thus arriving at the complete emancipation of the mind. I have often been asked to give an explanation of what Yoga is about and to provide indications as to the method and practice of Asanas and Pranayama. To meet with this demand and increasing interest, I decided to write this book, based on the practical experience of the great Indian Yogis and Sages, plus original Sanskrit writings on therapeutic yogic practices.

May Yoga prosper and bring peace to the world!

Sri Ananda

Contents

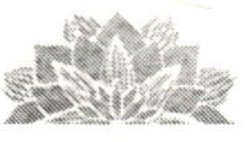

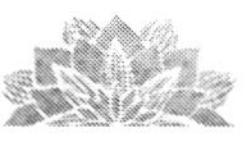

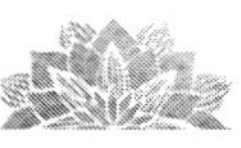

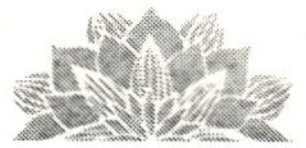

Section 1

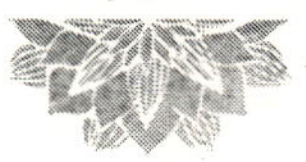

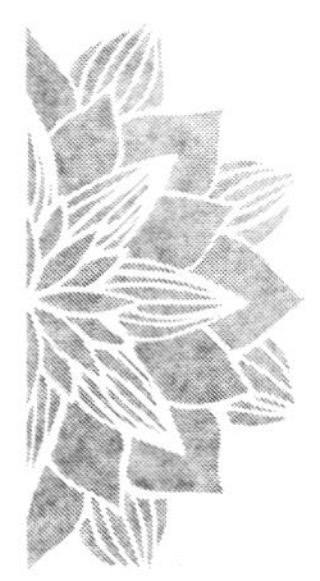

When this body
has been so
magnificently
and artistically
created by God,
it is only fitting
that we should
maintain it in
good health and
harmony by the
most excellent
and artistic
science of yoga.

Geeta Iyengar,
daughter of
B.K.S. Iyengar

1

In Search of Yoga

When I was a very young boy, my mother told me wonderful stories of the Yogis and their supernatural powers. Every day I would impatiently wait to hear another story about the Yogis, and would refuse to go to sleep unless I heard one, for it had become my great passion. My mother was a saintly woman, very gentle, pious and generous, with no limits to her charity. My father would say to her, 'If you go on giving everything away like that, there'll be nothing left for us and the children.' She used to reply fervently that God would take care of everything: and indeed He did. My mother not only helped the poor, but also all those who came to her for help, regardless of caste or religion, for she never disappointed anyone. This was to leave a deep and lasting impression on me, and become the torch lighting every moment of my life.

The very word 'Yogi' had a magical effect on me. Instead of going out to play with my friends, I spent my time reading all the books on Yoga I could lay my hands on. In some of them I read that the practice of Siddhasana (pose of an adept) and Sirshasana (head-stand) was the best way of achieving complete continence and the conversion of sexual energy into spiritual force, which will lead to the awakening of the Kundalini Shakti (coiled up cosmic energy lying dormant at the base of the spinal column).

It was then possible to develop such faculties as clairvoyance, telepathy, looking into the past and future, thought-reading and all sorts of occult powers. I had read and heard so much about the Yogis that Yoga had become my whole existence: I could not resist the temptation to try it out for myself.

During the summer holidays, I started to practise Siddhasana and Sirshasana all on my own, asking neither for advice nor guidance from a guru. I was convinced that the only person on earth to have discovered the secret of becoming a real Yogi was myself.

My sole thought was to practise Siddhasana and Sirshasana for hours on end, and to have the joy of acquiring supernatural powers. I was indifferent to the heat and cold, the pleasures and hardships of life, for I was living in a strange world of my own, convinced that these practices alone would suffice to make me a perfect Yogi: I fondly imagined that mere physical achievements would automatically lead to spiritual results.

The desire for mastery of the body and senses became so strong that I practised unceasingly. When I heard that salt, sweet things, and spicy or bitter foods were an impediment to spirituality, I gave them up without thinking twice. After a period of self-denied and discipline, however, the results were fairly slender. They were psychic, rather than spiritual as I had hoped, although this did help me develop determination and teach me to control my desires. I was bitterly disappointed and wondered why my Kundalini Shakti had not yet awoken. I also felt exhausted and disoriented, so I went to see and seek a guru. When I described my efforts to the guru I approached, he informed me that I had come in the nick of time, for had I continued, I would have landed in serious trouble.

I was also told that my incessant practicing without the guidance of a trained guru could have caused irreparable brain-damage due to an excessive influx of blood. He followed this with the observation that I should not be depressed or discouraged, however, and quoted a passage from the Upanishads:

> Those aspirants who allow their faults or failures to depress or discourage them unduly, make the way rougher and more difficult. But to recognize one's own errors in thoughts, feelings, words or deeds is the first condition of one's inner and outer progress.

He asked me to remain patient and explained that one should not except anything more than a slow evolution at the beginning.

The path of Yoga is not easy, every inch of ground has to be won against much resistance. The aspirant must be patient and firm to face difficulties, and obstacles of all sorts with a calm and serene spirit.

This experience taught me a lesson, and I realized that nobody should try to practise Yoga without the guidance of a guru. Later, I was to see just how true the ancient texts on Yoga are when they caution that the practice of Yoga required equilibrium, uniformity, order and discipline — as do all other human activities.

I subsequently realized that supernatural powers (*Siddhis*) are nothing but the fancies of human mind. A real Yogi or a true aspirant of Yoga does not aim at the enjoyment of these powers; his sole aspiration is to Self-realization. While I was following the

spiritual instructions of my Guru, he directed my interest towards research into therapeutic Yoga.

Yoga therapy is undoubtedly the surest means of preventing illness or helping to cure it. Illness is nature's way of letting us know that we should devote our attention to the repair of the body and the recovery of health. Our neglect of this is the result of ignorance. Knowledge and power are useless unless they benefit man's health. Good health is a gift of nature, and it is up to man to make a wholehearted effort to preserve it.

There are millions of men and women who are suffering. Thousands come and go without any knowledge of their internal disorders. Many of them appear to be strong and healthy, but are in fact suffering from physiological complaints. Constant work does not allow us to stop and think how to find a remedy for the harm that is wearing out our lives and those of future generations. A sedentary existence, over-eating, and unbalanced diet, over-work, tiring or badly chosen amusements: that is what the so-called modern, civilized life is made up of.

Modern man does not feel happy because he is dissatisfied with his way of life. If we dig deep, we realize that no form of happiness is possible for the individual as long as his physical and mental condition is less than perfect. The problem will only be solved when man enjoys sound health, remains pure in his thoughts, words and action, rises above a materialist attitude to life, and realizes that all his resources, indeed his life itself, should be used for the improvement of himself and his neighbour. Material wealth may perhaps ensure human well-being up to a point, but the real pivot on which life hinges remains good health.

Other Systems of Physical Exercise

I have studied various systems of physical exercise in an attempt to discover the best. There is no doubt that an active life with exercise in the open air and plenty of deep breathing is a necessity, but our idea of an active life or the aim of physical exercise is very specific. In general, what is meant by an 'active life' is in fact continuous work with few, if any, intervals of rest, while 'physical exercise' means the development and control of the muscles. People seek to develop prominent muscles, but fail to strengthen the cardiac muscle, lungs or nervous system. Whenever we exercise, we concentrate on the voluntary muscles, leaving aside the involuntary ones, so that toxins build up inside the body. Heavy perspiration and exhaustion after exercise are the proof of this.

The explanation is as follows: We make an extra-heavy demand for fresh blood without regard to the quantity of oxygen-rich purified blood required to meet this. A study of open-air games, sports and physical exercises shows that when we strain ourselves beyond our capacity, without medical supervision, the voluntary muscles of the arms, legs and other parts of the body will move at rapid intervals while exercising. This lead to high mortality rate for tissues and cells. The heart beats rapidly to meet the abnormal demand for fresh blood and the lungs are overworked, and so are the veins, for they are expected to carry impure blood from the body to the heart which pumps it to the lungs to be purified.

This rapid and continuous process causes great tension in the heart, lungs, veins and organs of the bloodstream in general; their force is thus reduced. It follows that the heart palpitates, the pulse races, the breathing is faster, while fatigue and perspiration exceed their normal limits. We are nevertheless convinced that this is the right thing for us to do to improve health. Even athletes or those who practise sport regularly should lie down and take a rest when in the

above state. Should they repeat the same schedule without taking heed of this, they will realize later that their resistance, endurance and powers of recuperation would have diminished, and the flexibility of youth would have given way to the stiffness of old-age. This explains why often athletes and famous wrestlers die of heart attacks — even in the prime of life.

The Discipline of Yoga

Those who practise only the Yoga postures and breathing exercises encounter the same difficulties as those resulting from physical exercises. One should know the laws of physiology and anatomy, because to adopt postures and do breathing exercises without the proper guidance can lead to serious consequences. One can, for example, stay in a posture for too long, carry out movements too quickly or repeat often hoping for spectacular progress and increased effects. It is a mistake to think that the more one perspires and tires oneself out, or the more aches and stiffness one feels, the better the results will be.

All organic life is a process of assimilation and elimination. Human life is no exception. The greater an individual's potential for assimilation and elimination, the greater the store of vital energy he possesses. The power of assimilation depends on that of relaxation, and the regenerative powers of the body cells. The metabolism is made up, on one hand, of the double process of the elimination of dead cells and other poisons in the organism, and on the other, of formation and continued growth of new cells. The development of the body does not only depend on the constant powers of multiplication, of living cells, but also on the degree of vital force, endurance and resistance they possess, plus their powers of recuperation. The greater the elasticity of these life cells, the higher their power of resistance and endurance. This explains why some people enjoy tremendous youthfulness, are resistant to illness, and can ward off premature old-age.

From my own experience and those who have worked under my guidance, it may be said that to obtain the maximum benefit from Asanas and Pranayama, complete mental and physical relaxation is absolutely essential. Physical effort engenders a demand for blood by the body. It is during relaxation that all the parts of the body are able to receive an adequate supply of oxygen-rich blood required. One should relax completely, therefore, both at the beginning and end of each Asana, and in addition, rhythmic breathing exercises should be performed.

Movements should be slow, well-balanced and uniform when carrying out postures. By slow, deliberate and regular movements, plus complete stretching at the required moment, we are able to bring deep-reaching pressure to bear on various parts of the body. If, on the other hand, our movements are quick, violent and abrupt, tissues and cells can neither be completely contracted, nor fully relaxed. Excessive effort should be carefully avoided; postures should not be prolonged beyond the time alloted, and, above all, we should relax the moment we begin to feel tired.

There are other, generally unknown, aspects of the Yoga method: these are the *counter-movements*. They should be performed after the various Asanas. They help to avoid convulsions, constriction, stiffness, and even pain provoked by the postures.

By following this method, even those who are mentally and physically exhausted will feel light, active and restored. It is not the Yoga system alone that counts, but the technique as well. This determines, to a great extent, the proper functioning of the different systems of the human body.

The Kriyas (techniques of internal purification):

The most widely known are the *dhauti, neti* and *basti*.

(a) *Dhauti* is the purification of the abdomen and stomach.
This is not simply swallowing a strip of material four fingers wide and five metres long. It should first be dipped in a bowl of water and water squeezed out. Then one of the ends is put into the mouth and swallowed inch-by-inch before being removed. This is how cleansing of the stomach and abdomen should be performed. Many people imagine that the Yogis remove their intestines and wash them, whereas they are simply carrying out *dhauti*.

(b) *Neti* is the flushing or cleansing of the nose.
There are two ways of doing this: the first is to take a bowl or glass of warm water, dip the nose in it and slowly breathe in the water through the nostrils. The water will automatically trickle down into the throat and be evacuated through the mouth.

The second is to use a string. This should be extremely soft and tightly-woven, and some eight inches (20 cms) long. The end should be stiffened with bees' wax. The string should be completely immersed in water, before being put into one nostril while the other is held closed with a finger. The string is then inhaled successively in deep breaths. Once it is felt at the back of the throat, it is taken between the index finger and thumb, very gently to avoid pain, then drawn out of the mouth and moved back and forth to thoroughly cleanse the nostril. The same is done for the other nostril.

(c) *Basti* is the washing of the intestines.
Provided one knows how to isolate the recto-abdominal muscles and open the sphincter at will, it is possible to draw water through the colon by slowly contracting the rectum. By giving the abdominal muscles a good shake, the water may be expelled immediately.

Many people are tempted to perform these various internal purification Kriyas to avoid illness, rather than practising the Asanas and Pranayama, in the belief that they will thus obtain better results. *We should not forget, however, that the Asanas and Pranayama, when performed correctly are more efficient than the various Kriyas. These can in fact be dispensed with completely, since they are very tricky, complicated and dangerous, and have in some cases proved harmful. Unless one practises them under the guidance of an expert familiar with their advantages and disadvantages, one should leave them well alone.*

Conclusion

My continuous research, plus direct experience at various yoga institutes, along with encounters with real Yogis and sages has led me to the conclusion that the Yoga method is the best discipline. It incorporates movements executed with a clearly defined end in view. It prevents loss of energy and promotes a balanced organism. Yoga ensures perfect health, plus the equilibrium and harmony that lead to happiness, peace and good spirits.

With regard to its physical aspects, the Yoga is both a curative and a preventive measure. As preventive therapy it is unequalled, whilst as a remedy it has proved to be helpful in the case of almost all known physical ailments — even those that have reached a critical stage. This particular method teaches man how to live a healthy, natural and normal life. If this way of life is followed correctly, it is beneficial both to the individual and to the world at large. The accent is put on a return to natural habits, in preference to those that result from an artificial lifestyle. The method not only acts on the physical body — caring for its well-being and strength — but helps also to preserve its natural state of good health. It aims at the coordination between mind and body, and man's harmonious evolution.

If we wish to possess perfect health, be immune to illness and live a long life; if we seriously wish to discover a method that enables us to maintain our health and recuperate our forces; if we are looking for real development of the muscles and not just their external appearance; if we want to stave off old age and delay death; in a word, if we want to make our lives happy, then we should follow the original Yoga method, for it is complete and rational, both from the point of view of hygiene and that of spiritual evolution. It satisfies the body, mind and soul simultaneously.

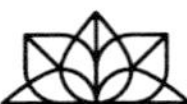 THE ORIGINS OF YOGA

Although increasingly more interest is being taken in Yoga by the West, there is still a great deal of mistrust, prejudice and many misconceptions about it.

It is a great pity that much of the published works on yoga give neither a clear idea of what Yoga is, nor provide any detailed knowledge on the subject. I would like to dispense with the erroneous ideas on Yoga and present the living truth about it.

Generally speaking, people in the West equate superstitions and unusual practices, still seen in some part of India with Yoga or spiritualism.

The origins of such superstitions reach back to successive invasions of India by foreign hordes; person of different races, tongues, beliefs and cultures settled here bringing with them many primitive ideas and superstitions most of which have gradually died out. Some have persisted, however, perpetuated by ignorance and lack of education. The essential truth remained deeply engraved in the consciousness of the evolved or highly cultured Hindus, who were able to guide those capable of following them. Superstitions and peculiar practices of the ignorant have no place either in Yoga or in Hindu spiritualism.

Some see Yoga as a kind of philosophy or religion, preaching a selfish introversion and the neglect of duties to family and society.

Yoga is not a religion. It is a philosophy of life based on certain psychological facts, and its aim is the development of a perfect balance between the body and the mind that permits union with the divine, i.e., a perfect harmony between the individual and the cosmos. Yoga does not always imply a retreat from the world, for the great Gurus and Sages of India, the founders of Yoga, were family-men who instructed their sons in the art of Self-knowledge. All the sacred writings of India (the *Vedas*, the *Upanishads*, the *Puranas* and the *Tantras*) are full of exploits by men and women of all castes, creeds and religions; people from all walks of life who arrived at the highest degree of knowledge through the discipline of Yoga — while carrying on their various occupations.

Scriptures on Yoga declare that the aim of human life is dedicated service of humanity, free from self-interest. The *Bhagavad Gita* tells us that 'the Yoga of action is superior to the Yoga of renunciation'. The great spiritual leaders of India have also drawn their inspiration from the *Vedas* and *Upanishads*.

What Are The Holy Scriptures

There are four *Vedas* (the word '*veda*' means 'knowledge'): the *Rig-Veda, Yajur-Veda, Sama-Veda* and *Atharva-Veda*. They contain not only the religious, philosophical and cultural ideas of the Hindus, but also the first fruits of a civilization. The *Vedas* are taken to be divine word itself, and not the work of man. We must understand them, not as writings, but as the sum of divine Knowledge. The wisdom of the *Vedas* is not limited to that of one particular individual; it is impersonal and as eternal as God.

The philosophical section of the *Vedas* is contained in the *Upanishads*, they form the basis for various systems of thought. The word '*upanishad*' means literally 'teaching that destroys ignorance'.

The *Puranas* are a series of 18 epic poems recording the legendary lives and deeds of divine incarnations.

The *Tantras* (whose name is derived from the root *tan* 'to spread'; *tatri* or *tantri* means 'origins of knowledge') provide a way towards the realization of the Supreme Goal. The *Bhagavad Gita*, the Song of the Lord, belongs to the epic poem *Mahabharata* and contains teachings of the kind found in the *Upanishads*.

People also tend to confuse Yoga with the practices of the fakirs, or with spiritualism and other practices ending in 'ism'. They are amazed by the contortions and abnormal powers they take for Yoga. Everything they fail to understand seems senseless to them; anything that is outside their range of intellectual experience seems stupid, and if modern science has no answer to it, it must be fake. To be fair, one must admit that their attitude is almost inevitable, for they are unable to raise their thoughts upwards, so that these remain on a low level and lack objectivity. They judge everything according to their own limited knowledge, thus considerably reducing the field of their experience.

I am often asked if Yogis are able to perform feats, contortions and other feats, such as stopping the heart from beating at will, drinking acid, swallowing poison, chewing glass, driving a knife through the tongue, lying on a bed of nails, being buried alive for several weeks, walking over fire, doing a disappearing act and so on. The next question is whether I am able to perform them too! Sometimes, people may be seen in the streets of India exhibiting the mastery and dominance they exercise over their body by doing contortions and performing bizarre tricks. They draw large crowds and thus earn a little money: such people are called fakirs.

There are also ambitious people who develop the power of concentration through the practice of Yoga so that they may exploit certain situations to their own advantage.

In fact, neither health nor spiritual activities require such practices. Those who are attracted by the thought of obtaining supra-normal powers, and thus carry out such practices, are generally weak, unintelligent and spiritually unaware.

Such practices are not a part of Yoga, and such people should not be confused with Yogis. Real yogis do not sit by the street side to titillate the curiosity of passersby. They are wise, saintly men who live in the highest realm of spiritual existence.

Yoga is the experience of complete peace of mind and self-knowledge. It trains the mind psychologically and increases the power of perception. Due to concentration, Yoga helps us perceive the subtle realities of life, illuminating our existence and moral sense. It directs our lives and spiritual aspirations towards their perfect self-expression and an accomplishment where knowledge unites the knower with that which is known.

The tradition of Yoga was born in India several thousand years ago, founded by the Rishis and Maharshis, great saints and sages. They were genuine Yogis who had complete mastery over mind and body, and also what are known as supernatural powers and arts. They recognized that life had its limits, and brought with it inevitable pain and suffering due to its duality and the countless

illusions. They realized that there was a meaning to life and some purpose beyond suffering. They were convinced that there was a way of escaping the tragic problems of life. Their efforts to find the truth bore fruit, for they crossed the frontiers of the mind, the limits of the senses and of intellectual reasoning. Philosophers and religions all over the world assure us that there comes a time when the human mind is able to transcend both the limits of the senses and the power of reasoning. The Sages saw the most secret truths of life, thanks to their supersensuous perceptions, arrived at through the concentration of the powers of the mind. They were moved also by the suffering they saw and wanted to deliver man from ignorance and set him on the road to freedom. The great Yogis gave rational interpretations of their experiences and brought within everyone's reach a practical, scientifically prepared method. It was so devised that any human being could understand it and follow the real paths of life through these experiences leading to the final goal: the realization of the Self (illumination).

To begin with, this knowledge only existed in monasteries, ashrams, the caves of the Himalayas and in the heart of deep forests. It was taught by a guru to those who were suitable to receive it. They were called *shishyas* (disciples). Later on, Yoga spread among the common people. The science developed in several ways. Among the most important works on this subject are the *Yoga Sutra* or *Aphorisms of Patanjali* with a commentary by Vyasa.

Today, Yoga is no longer restricted to a privileged minority of hermits: it has taken its place in our everyday lives.

WHAT IS YOGA?

Generally speaking, the average person's level of consciousness is fairly low. He is enslaved to life and lives on false hopes and illusions. He spends his life in ignorance, experiencing joy and sorrow, success and failure, love and grief, without ever really coming to the ultimate realization. The great mass of humanity allows itself to be led and dominated by the senses and commit errors which they subsequently regret. They delude themselves by looking for peace, happiness and self-accomplishment through the pleasures of the senses. It is quite normal for the human mind to want to discover the underlying facts and principles of nature by means of a physical experience. We notice straightaway that the experiences we have on a physical level are only temporary, superficial and illusory, since our senses are limited. It is of course a help to know about material things to achieve material ends, but such knowledge cannot show us the true aim of existence.

Modern science provides us with leisure, comfort and an easier material existence; but it does not give us peace of mind and inner calm. There are so many examples of people who have everything they need materially, and yet unhappy, restless and tormented.

The purpose of life should be sought in the depths of the soul, by means of experience, hope, faith, peace of mind and spiritual wisdom. Things experienced on a spiritual level are both permanent and true. It is at this moment that illusion falls away and Truth shines in all its splendour.

Just as an image cannot be reflected in a dusty mirror or crystal bowl full of muddy water, so also the mind of an average person is habitually obscured by ignorance, illusion and egocentricity.

The various Yogas present the means allowing man to lift the veil of ignorance and illusion (Maya), so that the mind may reflect the light of the Ultimate Reality.

The word 'Yoga' comes from the Sanskrit root '*yug*' meaning 'to join'. It designates 'the joining of the lower human nature to the higher in such a manner as to allow the higher to direct the lower', or 'union with the Self'. It also signifies communion with the supreme Universal Spirit to obtain relief from pain and suffering.'

> One who controls his mind, intellect and ego, being absorbed in the spirit within him, finds fulfilment and internal bliss which is beyond the pale senses and reasoning.
>
> — *Bhagavad Gita*

The great sages of India had perfected several methods, each adapted to a different temperament, so that everyone may reach the goal according to his own mental and physical capacities. Although these Yoga methods appear to be different, their aim is the same: Self-realization. The main point is that all methods of Yoga teach discipline and self-control without which all yoga is useless.

THE VARIOUS SYSTEMS OF YOGA

By and large, there are four types of persons in the world: the intellectual, active, emotional and contemplative.

Those who are *intellectual* follow the way of *Jnana Yoga*, the way of wisdom and discernment.

Those who are *active* follow the way of *Karma Yoga*, the way of action and service rendered without selfish motives, e.g., Mahatma

Gandhi, who showed the world that one could find God by serving man.

Those who are *emotional* follow the way of *Bhakti Yoga*, the path of devotion and love, where the personality is dissolved and the individual becomes completely unselfish.

Those who attach the greatest importance to *contemplation* follow the path of *Raja Yoga*, i.e., the way designed to control and master the mind by mental concentration. Raja Yoga recommends suitable methods and the practice of postures and breathing control, called *Hatha-Yoga*, with a view to finding calm, mental balance and peace of mind. Bodily health is very important for mental growth; this is why Hatha-Yoga and Raja Yoga complement one another. They constitute the same process in the liberation of the spirit. Later on we shall present a detailed study of the Hatha-Yoga system.

There are many other Yogas: union with the divine power (Kundalini Yoga); mastery of thought through meditation (Dhyana Yoga); repetition of sacred recitations (Mantra Yoga); control of the will (Laya Yoga); control of the forces present in human nature (Shakti Yoga); use of symbolic gesture during meditation (Mudra Yoga); and realization of a mystic experience (Yantra Yoga).

All these variations belong to one of the four main Yogas, which sometimes seem so similar that it is difficult to distinguish one from another.

> Yoga is not for those who fast or torture their flesh, who sleep too much or keep awake, who work too much or don't work at all.
>
> — *Bhagavad Gita*

Extremes should be avoided: too much fasting or too little sleep weakens the body and is detrimental to the nervous system. If we practise moderation and discipline, balance our eating and sleeping habits along with our work and the time we spend awake, we shall reach perfect harmony with the Self. In this way Yoga banishes pain and misery. To achieve this perfect harmony and complete equilibrium, we must have absolute control of both mind and body.

> The Self cannot be known by one who is dull or restless, who is not strong, disciplined and self-controlled. Neither can it be known by much learning nor by reasoning. It can be known only through calmness of mind, through practice of Yoga and through meditation.
>
> — *Upanishads*

MENTAL ATTITUDE

Medical experiments and psychological research have shown that negative mental attitudes are dangerous and lead to illness. They may act either directly or indirectly, in the form of heart attacks or failures or illnesses which may be traced back to the accumulation of uninterrupted tension.

There are of course temorary ways of escaping, in the form of alcohol or tranquilizers, but such remedies are destructive, even though they may not be fatal. They accelerate the ageing process, and leave one depressed or demoralized, and lead, in the end, to serious illnesses.

In many cases, people worry habitually for no reason. They imagine things that have not happened and may never happen, e.g., that they will be ruined financially and left without a penny to live on; that they are ill or about to fall sick; they are frightened of being left on their own, of being alone, of growing old, etc.

It goes without saying that such people impute their state to material circumstances, and lead a hectic life, rather than admitting that such imaginary illnesses may be traced back to within themselves.

According to scientific research on Yoga carried out at the Lonavla centre in India, and by the medical scientists in the West, constant worry and prolonged grief provoke the formation of calculus stones, i.e., small stones in the gall-bladder or kidneys. Frustration and overwork lead to nervous exhaustion.

Alcohol, tobacco and a diet that is too greasy or contains too much salt often provoke hypertension, while unsatisfied desires, disheartenment, disappointment and despair produce a kind of stomach acidity that results in ulcers.

A sudden fright causes diarrhoea while frequent agitation brings on heart and varicose troubles. A state of anxiety may also be the cause of chronic constipation.

All this goes to show that mental energy, when used negatively, will sooner or later cause us to fall ill.

The moment we use mental energy positively, we change our attitude and outlook. A positive mental attitude, coupled with faith, sweep away all our doubts, so that we seem to possess an inner force that is great enough for us to overcome all our difficulties.

It is common knowledge among psychologists that a person's reaction to an event is more important than the event itself: when

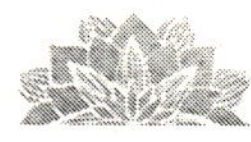

we look the facts in the face, however hard they may be, they are not as important as our attitude towards them. An event may overwhelm us mentally before we have even begun to get to grips with it. *One of the most powerful factors is to have confidence in oneself.*

When Yoga is practised correctly and conscienciously, it becomes a sure way of restoring balance, helping us to develop determination and resistance, and above all, to find serenity and inner peace.

POWER OF MIND

> 'If matter is mighty, thought is Almighty.'
>
> — *Swami Vivekananda*

We have noted earlier in the book that the body reacts to the slightest impulse from the mind. The opposite is also true: if the body is sick, the mind too falls ill, while a healthy body means a healthy mind. Similarly, if the mind is disturbed, the body will also be troubled. In general, those who are strong and healthy have a calm temperament, while the weak and unhealthy are easily annoyed. The influence of mind over body is, however, much greater than that of body over mind. Our evolution depends on whether we direct our thoughts positively or negatively, for an individual acts according to his thoughts and reaps the harvest of his actions.

Let us now examine the strong influence the mind has over body especially with regard to emotions. Emotions can be gentle or violent, positive or negative, and when emotions reach their height, we call them passions.

Anger, hate, jealousy, fear, despair, etc., are negative emotions. It is clear that the repercussions they have on the body are more or less far-reaching according to how intense they are. Frequent emotional upsets affect the whole of the nervous system and may result in illness. Repeated assaults on the nervous system are harmful to the endocrine glands and may lead to ageing and premature death.

Sometimes the most vigorous constitutions are paralysed by overwhelming fear, and the strongest may be undermined by worries. During a fit of rage, we may lose control over our nerves with resulting actions that may be regretted later on.

There are also positive emotions, such as hope and confidence. They promote the wellbeing of the nervous system and make the body healthy. Love, joy and happiness bring peace to the mind and make us optimistic.

Nevertheless, when emotions are sudden and violent, whether they be positive (joy) or negative (sorrow), they may be detrimental, for they create an inner upheaval which may be fatal.

This proves that the mind is strong enough to influence the body in every possible way. It is obvious that physical exercise can never produce the expected results unless supported by mental discipline. How can we expect to build up good health, a strong nervous system and the proper functioning of our endocrine glands if we allow our mind to wander direction less? How can we have a peaceful, vigorous mind if our brain is beset by constant preoccupations?

This is why all the ancient books on Yoga, such as *Yoga Shastra*, *Hatha-Yoga Pradeepika* and *Yoga-Sutra* by Patanjali state that the '*Yamas*' (mental discipline), and the '*Niyamas*' (mental purification), should be practised first, and only then followed by the '*Asanas*'

The *Yamas* and *Niyamas* are principles of good conduct, which if followed correctly, bring supreme peace of mind. The individual is then freed of all violent emotion; he develops faith in himself, preserving an indestructible optimism and clear-sightedness.

- *Ahimsa* (non-violence), *Satya* (truth), *Asteya* (non-stealing), *Brahmacharya* (chastity) and *Aparigraha* (non-covetousness) are *Yamas*, i.e., rules of good conduct for society and the individual.

- *Saucha* (purity of body and mind), *Santosa* (contentment), *Tapas* (self-discipline and austerity), *Svadhyaya* (study of scriptures) and *Ishwara Pranidhana* (worshipping God and contemplation are the *Niyamas*, i,e., rules for self-purification related to personal discipline.

Rigorous practice of the Yamas and Niyamas is absolutely essential for those following the spiritual path. Those who turn to Yoga regarding it as nothing more than physical health and mental peace, or as a method of healing, may practise the Yamas and Niyamas to keep their minds healthy and to augment their inner force. In everyday terms, this means that to practise them on a modest scale is quite sufficient, requiring only a change in one's daily habits.

When our mental energy or consciousness is disciplined, we can direct it to any part of the body, and immediately find a reaction: the sensation of feeling better. This is due to the abundant flow of blood sent to that part of the body. In this way we are gradually able to fortify and animate all the areas of the body.

After all, illness is nothing other than the expression of the unequal distribution of vital forces throughout the human body. Whenever vital energy is unbalanced, the body's stability is disturbed, and we fall victim to all kinds of irregularities. This state is called 'illness'. If the currents of vital force are consciously and equally directed to all parts of the body, we can recover by achieving equilibrium and regaining perfect mental and physical harmony.

Both the prevention and healing of illness should begin in the mind. 'Prevention is better than cure.'

YOGA IN OUR TIME

> The younger, the old, the extremely aged, even the sick and the infirm obtain perfection in Yoga by constant practice. Success in Yoga is obtained by mere theoretical study, or talking about it or reading the sacred texts. Constant practice alone is the secret of its success.
>
> — *Hatha Yoga Pradeepika*

> Through constant practices of Yoga, one can overcome all difficulties and eradicate all weaknesses. Pain can be transmuted into bliss, sorrow into joy, failure into success and sickness into perfect health. Determination, patience, persistence lead us to the goal.
>
> — *Bhagavad Gita*

Basically human evolution takes place on three different planes: physical, mental and spiritual.

Nature has enabled physical life to reach full maturity. The harmony of matter and life-energy have arrived at their accomplishment. It is only inertia of the physical body and troubles provoked by bad distribution of vital energy often create an obstacle to the development of man's latent potentiality.

Following the body, it is the mind through which we enable our physical life to evolve towards elevated aims. Mental life, in the present times, is not, however, fully developed in the case of most people. For the majority, the mind is inactive and sometimes even retarded. The most remarkable manifestations of the mind are only reached in exceptional cases. The main obstacle to the development of the inner life is persistent ignorance of the nature of the human mind. It is at this point that Yoga intervenes to show us the secrets of nature that lead to a spiritual life.

All the experiences of Yoga confirm the fact that the mind, like the body, is nothing more than an instrument to be used in helping us reach a state of super-consciousness, a state in which only pure knowledge and beatitude exist.

Science depends on knowledge that is enlarged, revalidated by experiments, analysis and consistent results, whereas Yoga relies on direct perception and experience. It is a way of perfecting oneself and developing one's being. Yoga brings about individual evolution much more quickly than the slow process of nature.

Yoga should be taken as a method to obtain perfect health and maintain the physiological harmony of the body, as well as to achieve a state of mental perfection by progressing spiritually, as a result of complete self-control.

We may conclude from this that Yoga is universal; it is a path on which all those who have determination may start, whatever their age, social status, belief or religion. Yoga does not contain any mysteries and is accessible to everyone. *There is just one condition: It must be practised regularly under proper guidance.*

Yoga brings hope and self-confidence to all those who are disappointed by their materialistic life or are inextricably bound up in all sorts of problems. It casts light on the practical and psychological side of life's problems and those of our spiritual conscience. It is a unique method for us to allow our personality to unfold to its fullest extent.

Yoga teaches us to live reasonably and avoid squandering our energy; it also shows us how to exercise self-control and preserve a positive attitude towards life. This way Yoga leads us towards universal love, for it is by love alone that we may create a brotherhood of man between the various nations of the world.

MEDITATION

> Sthira-Sukham Asanam
> (comfortable and firm position)
>
> — *Patanjali Sutra, 46*

Dhyana or the *state of meditation* is obtained when the mind is trained to concentrate on an outer or inner object, long enough for all distractions to be eliminated, and when the stream of thought flows in a single direction without interruption towards a definite subject.

During meditation, the body is silently resting so that thought is absorbed into *Prana* (vital force). As in dreamless sleep, so here too, the only sign of life is breathing. The hypothalamus recharges its energy during meditation, as it does during sleep. We may deduce from this that whereas sleep is a compensating form of rest, meditation is a conscious one, and hence contains important therapeutic characteristics.

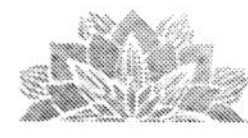

Meditation helps us to rid ourselves of emotional conflict, inner discord and psychological tension. It completely purifies the mind and frees it from unconscious obstructions. Meditation enables the inner light to manifest itself. This is responsible for the awakening of Self-awareness, hence one may penetrate to the very centre of life's highest values.

The subject of meditation may be the Supreme-Self, pure existence or Universal Value. The commonest traditional method consists in concentrating one's attention on an object of personal value or a universal symbol.

For example, a Hindu will choose one of the divinities that he is familiar with: Shiva, Vishnu, Krishna, Kali or some other divine incarnation. He may also choose the sacred syllable *'Aum' (Om)*, considered a symbol of the Absolute in the Hindu religion.

For a Buddhist, subjects of meditation may be statues of Buddha, the Lotus or the Wheel (Mandala).

A Christian will choose the image of Christ on the Cross.

The Star of David in Judaism or the Crescent of the first quarter of the new moon for Islam, also serve subjects for meditation.

To sum up, we may say that each person, according to his faith, will choose an elevated thought or spiritual symbol upon which he prefers to meditate. The aim here is not to enter in detail into all the various techniques of meditation, but simply to give an outline of the practices in use at present, to help those who aspire to the spiritual path.

Meditation Depends on 3 Main Physiological Factors

(1) A comfortable and firm posture must be adopted, otherwise meditation is impossible; a firm posture means to hold oneself in such a way that one is conscious of the body. A slightest discomfort in posture will be a constant distraction to the mind; one should therefore choose the position that allows one to remain still for a long time without feeling discomfort.

(2) The spine and head should be kept very straight, but without being strained. All the ancient texts on Yoga insist on the necessity of keeping the spine straight during meditation to avoid pressure on the abdominal organs, for this leads to a stooping position that brings on constipation and lays the way for many other disorders. There is another reason for holding oneself straight; the nerves in the coccyx and sacrum receive a more copious blood-supply, which helps to revitalise them.

(3) In meditation posture, the expenditure of muscular energy decreases, so that the movement of the heart and lungs slows down; the production of carbonic gas is at its lowest; breathing becomes very light, almost abdominal, so that one can scarcely feel it. Under such conditions, the mind is almost completely protected from the distractions caused by physical movement, and can therefore be directed inwardly in complete tranquillity.

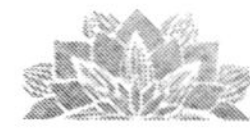

THE NADIS, CHAKRAS AND KUNDALINI

> The Nadis are like the fibres of a lotus, and being supported by the vertebral column, spread downwards.
>
> — *Shiva Samhita, 11-17*

Among the countless *nadis*, the three most important are situated along the spinal column: the *Ida* on the left side, the *Pingala* on the right, and the *Sushuma* in the middle.

According to the Yogis, the Ida and Pingala are the main channels along which the afferent and efferent currents flow. One carries sensations to the brain, and the other flows from the brain to the body. The *Sushumna* is a hollow channel along which the *Kundalini* flows upwards. The *Vedas* call it the channel of enlightened vigilance or *Brahmanadi*.

During meditation, the Yogis direct their attention to certain subtle centres called Chakras. These are responsible for the equal distribution of energy to the body.

The seven main Chakras are: the *Muladhara*, at the base of the spine; the *Svadhishthana*, between the navel and the genital organs; the *Manipura*, in the area of the navel; the *Anahata* in the heart region; the *Vishuddha* in the throat with the thyroid gland; the *Ajna* between the eyebrows; and the *Sahasrara* on top of the head.

Kundalini is cosmic energy symbolized by a sleeping serpent coiled in the *Muladhara*. When the Kundalini, or latent energy, is aroused as a result of the appropriate postures, Pranayama exercises and meditation, it makes its way upwards via the *Sushumna*, passing through the *Chakras* one after the other. Whenever it reaches a new *Chakra*, the Yogi attains a higher state of consciousness.

Faculties may be acquired, such as clairvoyance, telepathy, knowledge of past and future, ability to read other people's thoughts, as well as many other occult powers, depending on the Chakra upon which one is meditating. The Yogi does not stop at this, however, for although he possesses all these occult powers, he brushes them aside, aspiring to the highest degree of knowledge: the realization of the Supreme-Self, the Ultimate Truth.

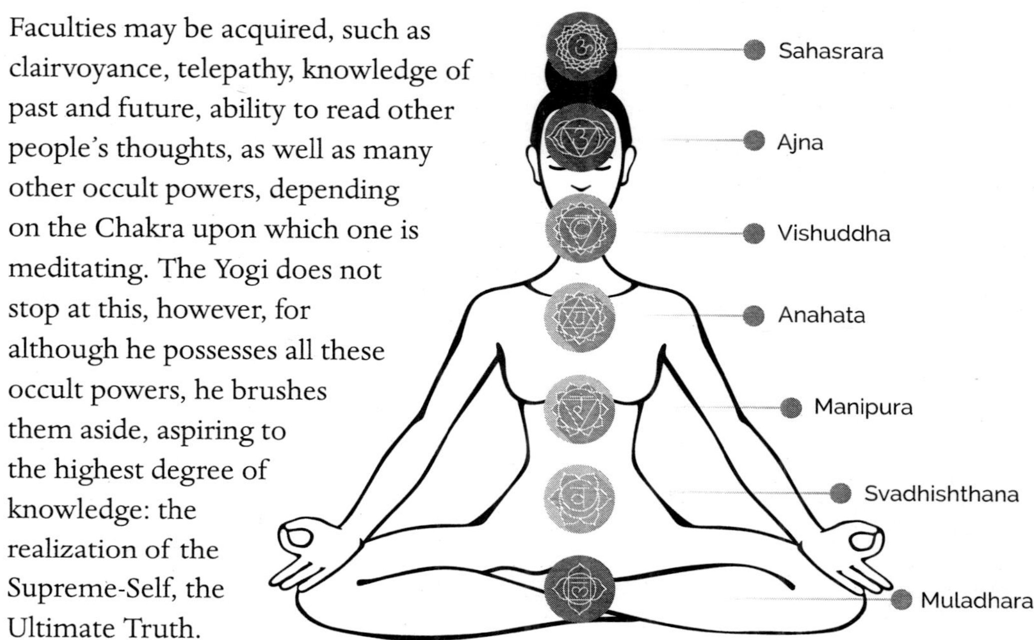

Once the Yogi practising Raja Yoga has directed the Kundalini by the power of concentration to the seventh Chakra, the *Sahasrara* (the seat of pure-consciousness), and has united himself to it, he has attained the true goal of meditation: the state of super consciousness or *Samadhi*.

N.B.: One should never attempt this without proper guidance, otherwise the results will be disastrous.

Experience of Yoga shows us that consciousness is responsible for certain vibrations that pass through the body. Individually, we can only raise our degree of consciousness in proportion to the level of resistance in the nervous system. If we raise the vibrations too quickly, the body and the whole of the nervous system may be destroyed by currents arriving too suddenly and in excess. This is explained by the fact that the body is not prepared for the high tension of cosmic forces. It is also the reason why it is absolutely

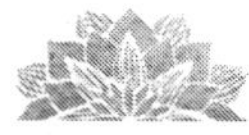

essential to make the body healthy and resistant by practising suitable Yoga Asanas and Pranayama exercises. The control of physical conditions enables all bodily functions to be subordinated to the mind, so that we are freed from desires and passions. The mind then becomes immobile and can be directed inwardly in total calm, to attain complete Illumination.

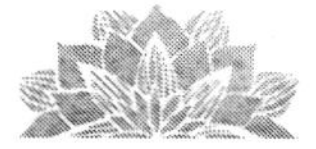

Section 2

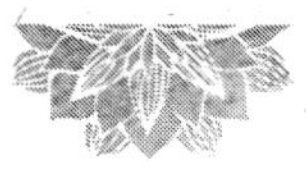

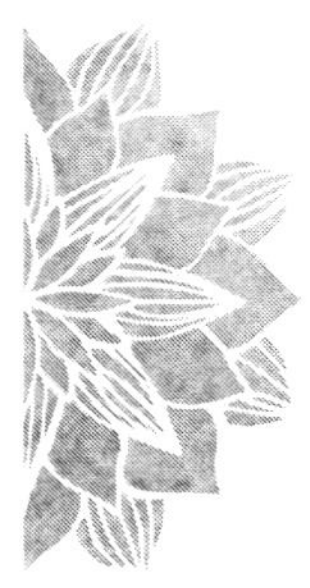

Understanding
without practice
is better than
practice without
understanding.
Understanding with
practice is better
than understanding
without practice.
Residing in your
true nature is better
than understanding
or practice.

Upanishads

2

Hatha Yoga

> Mastery of the body and breath are an undoubted aid to those concerned with their spiritual evolution. For by having full control over the physical condition, the body becomes calm, allowing the mind to be directed inwardly more easily in perfect tranquillity, to achieve a higher spiritual level.
>
> — *Hatha Yoga Pradeepika*

WHAT IS HATHA YOGA?

Hatha-Yoga is a discipline whose aim is to ensure perfect health by physical and mental purification through the control of the mind and body. It allows man to reach his full potential, an objective which may only be achieved if there is balance and harmony between the body and mind. The power of concentration can then develop, loading to the realization of the Self.

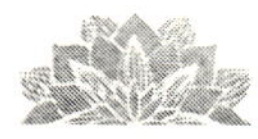

The power of concentration is the greatest strength to awaken the mind and animate the body. When properly directed, it illuminates facts for us and brings the desired results.

> There is no limit to the power of the human mind. The more concentrated it is the more power is brought to bear on one point.
>
> The powers of the mind are like rays of light dissipated; when they are concentrated they illumine.
>
> — *Swami Vivekananda*

According to ancient Sanskrit texts, '*Ha*' means 'sun', i.e., positive energy, and '*Tha*' the moon, i.e., negative energy; the word 'Yoga' comes from the Sanskrit root '*Yug*' meaning 'to link, join or unite'; it also signifies a yolk.

'Hatha Yoga' is the meeting of two forces animating the human body, i.e., the union of positive energy (symbolized by the sun) and negative energy (symbolized by the moon) plus a perfect balance. Mastery of these two currents and complete equilibrium between them will keep us in perfect health.

Hatha Yoga is composed of three inseparable factors:
- Control of the mind;
- Pranayama (control and regulation of breath);
- Asanas (bodily postures).

These three factors are so closely linked that one without the others loses its value. It has been observed that we often live only one aspect of our lives, and remain ignorant of the others. A man with a brilliant mind may appear quite remarkable, even if it is housed in a sick, stunted body, while a magnificently developed body may often contain a feeble intelligence; this situation is unable to last long, and breaks down in the end due to imbalance.

To live harmoniously, the body and mind should be developed in a balanced way, through Pranayama and the Asanas. It is possible — perhaps unconsciously — to move the body or keep it immobile, then to breathe, but we cannot achieve control of the breathing or the body unless we are consciously aware of them. It is the fact that we are consciously aware of what we are doing that allows us to bring the body and mind into harmony and create the required and essential equilibrium. Hatha Yoga shows us how these three factors should be combined. For unless they are practised in conjunction, there will be no therapeutic effect.

It Asanas are performed in collaboration with the mind and proper breathing, the effect is almost immediate. The power of concentrated thought is so great that once we know how to direct it to each part of the body, it helps us to animate and revitalize the whole organism, which then functions under the control of the consciousness.

The main object of Pranayama is to acquire mastery of the vital forces acting within the body. It also helps to ensure the arousal and liberation of the latent psychic energy in the organism. With the aid of Pranayama, we can transform cosmic into human energy, thus maintaining the equilibrium of forces within the body.

The Asanas are useful, not only to revive the body, strengthen the nervous system and regenerate the glands, but also to cure physical and mental illness. They bring the human body under complete control of the mind.

The Asanas and Pranayamas are an effective means of promoting the harmonious development of the body, an efficient, powerful instrument of spiritual progress. Regular practice of Asanas and Pranayamas combined with control of the mind, combats negative elements such as ignorance, laziness, inertia, and over-excitement, as well as increases will power. Hatha Yoga should be the starting-point for all forms of Yoga, for a healthy body is the

absolute prerequisite for all human endeavour, whether physical or intellectual. Think of the proverb *Mens sana in corpore sano* — 'a healthy mind in a healthy body'.

It has been observed that even the mystics who neglected their bodies experienced great physical suffering, i.e., various illnesses, imbalance and premature death.

Deep spiritual experiences produce exhaustion of the nervous system, because they give rise to a highly emotional state. Unless the mystics have robust nerves and a trained body, they are not always able to transform their experience into creative energy. This explains why control of the nervous system and vital energy is absolutely essential.

The first and most important step is to train and develop the body to its fullest. This is only possible with the help of Asana and Pranayama exercises. The system is known as Hatha Yoga.

The Hatha Yoga method is quite unique; it shows us how to recuperate and store the largest amount of Prana, enables us to distribute Prana equally throughout the body and ensures the proper functioning of all the systems of the organism. The Asanas have been developed over the course of centuries. They are highly beneficial to health, and the part played by them in the preservation of the vital force is indisputable. When practised regularly, they ensure agility, balance, endurance, great vitality, and defence against illness. The Asanas eliminate tiredness and calm the nerves, so that sleep becomes truly restful.

They also bring mental balance by preventing the mind stay focused. These are the main advantages of Yoga exercises.

> When the mind and body are working together harmoniously due to Yoga discipline, we can find calm and peace of mind at every moment.
>
> — *Bhagavad Gita*

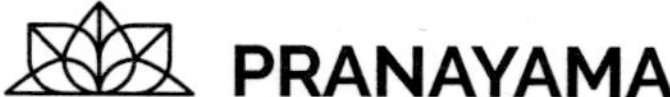

PRANAYAMA

What is Pranayama?

The Sanskrit word *Prana* means 'vital force' or 'cosmic energy'. It also signifies 'life' or 'breath'. '*Ayama*' means the control of the *Prana*. Hence Pranayama means the control of the vital force by concentration and regulated breathing.

The vital force or primordial life-force (*Prana*) manifests itself in the body as a respiratory function. It is the force motivating several other involuntary functions, among them the blinking of the eyes and even yawning. The *Prana* not only ensures the proper functioning of the body (including the glandular system), but is also the regulator and animator of the psyche. It is, in every sense of the word, the breath of the Spirit. Pranayama therefore provides a remedy for several of the physical and psychic disturbances of which modern man is the victim.

According to the *Yoga Shastra* (ancient Sanskrit texts on Yoga), the universe is composed of two substances: The *Akasa* (ether) and the *Prana* (cosmic energy). Everything which has a form, or is the result of a combination, evolves out of the *Akasa*. It is the *Akasa* that becomes the air, liquids, solids, the human body, animals, plants, etc. Everything we can touch, all the forms that we see, everything that exists, is due to the *Akasa*. It is so subtle that we cannot perceive it, for it is only visible once it has taken form. The power by which it is transformed into the universe is *Prana*.

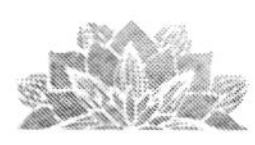

Everything we call energy or force evolves out of *Prana*. In all forms of life, from the highest to the lowest, the *Prana* is present as a living force. In the West, scientists say that the universe is full of energy which corresponds in fact to *Prana*. All force is based on *Prana*; it is the origin of movement, gravity, magnetism, physical action, the nerve currents and the force of thought. Without *Prana* there can be no life, for it is the soul of all force and energy. It is found in the air, water and food. *Prana* is the vital force inside each living being, and thought is the highest and most refined action of *Prana*.

As we breathe, the movement of the lungs inhaling air is the expression of *Prana*. Pranayama is not simply the breathing, but the control of the muscular force activating the lungs.

The organism can easily absorb *Prana* through fresh air in the process of breathing; there are three kinds of breathing: normal, deep, and controlled Yogic breathing.

With normal breathing, we absorb a normal quantity of Prana. When we breathe deeply, the volume absorbed increases, and with controlled Yogic breathing we are able to store a large quantity of *Prana* in the brain and nervous centres. It may be used in emergency, i.e., moments of life where we have to overcome unexpected difficulties. This store of *Prana* also builds up our resistance to contagious diseases.

In contrast to the above, if we breathe irregularly, haphazardly without thinking, the supply of *Prana* will gravitate towards a single part of the body and hence the equilibrium of the *Pranic* current will be disturbed, provoking a number of disorders within.

The practice which incorporates the control of *Prana* through the concentration of thought and regular breathing is called 'Pranayama'. It is through Pranayama that each part of the body can be filled with *Prana*. Once one is capable of performing it, one is master of the body and can dominate illness and suffering. One can indeed acquire control on another person's body. In the West, for example, followers of faith healing, spiritism, hypnotism and mental therapy, try to collect and control *Prana* unconsciously. They call it a 'force' and use it to cure illness. Their will-power is directed, through faith, towards the awakening of the patient's dormant *Prana*, i.e., they have the ability to bring their will power to a certain degree of vibration that may be transmitted to another person, arousing similar vibrations in him. So in fact, genuine healing is arrived at through *Prana*. It is perfectly true that people have been cured in such a way, even at a distance, but this method is not as easy to perform as is generally thought. For every genuine case there are hundreds of frauds.

According to ancient texts on Yoga, there is a deep affinity between *Prana* and mental force, for it is *Prana* that keeps the mind and body alive. It is only when we succeed in mastering *Prana* and directing it at will that we can hope to animate and develop a healthy body and a mind, free from all illness. *Prana is accumulated where our mind in concentrated.*

Thought is the absolute master controlling *Prana*-energy. Just as we are able to make ourselves ill and weak by negative thinking, so may we cure ourselves by expelling bad thoughts and replacing them with positive ones. Thus it becomes easy to avoid problems, by increasing and maintaining our vital force through Pranayama.

Pranayama is, therefore, the essential factor in our lives. It is a basic necessity for safeguarding our health. An abundant inhaling of *Prana* fills the body with new energy. It strengthens the heart, the organ which pumps blood and distributes *Prana* via the bloodstream to the smallest cells in the body.

Yoga Shastra tells us that *Prana* in the air we breathe fulfils several functions in the human body. Each of these has a special name:

- *Prana* (here the general term takes on a specific meaning) circulates in the area around the heart and controls breathing.
- *Apana* circulates in the lower regions of the abdomen and controls execretory functions (urine and faeces).
- *Samana* stimulates the gastric juices, thus facilitating digestion.
- *Udana* remains in thoractic cage, controls the absorbtion of air and food.
- *Vyana* spreads throughout the body and distributes the energy from food and breath.
- *Naga* relieves abdominal pressure by provoking eructation.
- *Kurma* controls the eyelids to prevent foreign bodies from entering and strong light from harming the eyes.
- *Krkara* prevents certain substances from rising into the nasal cavities or descending into the throat, causing sneezing and coughing.
- *Devadutta* ensures the absorption of extra oxygen into a tired body, provokes yawning.
- *Dhanamjaya* remains in the body, even after death, and sometimes causes the corpse to swell.

In conclusion, we can say that deep and regular breathing is absolutely essential for the health of the nervous system, brain and endocrine glands.

Owing to the artificial conditions in which we live, our breathing tends to be haphazard and irregular. The body does not take in enough *Prana*. The entire nervous system is harmed and the endocrine glands no longer function properly. The body begins to lose its force and vigour and there is a constant feeling of tiredness and depression. An inadequate supply of *Prana* also weakens the heart.

It is noticeable that to a great extent a person's physical condition depends on the regularity of breathing; even highly emotional states and passions are reflected in the breathing pattern.

During periods of emotional upset, such as depression, distress, or melancholia, breathing becomes very slow and irregular, but during fits of rage, agitation and nervousness, it becomes rapid, superficial and disordered. The result of such continual irregularities in breathing is that we not only harm the nervous system, but impede the proper functioning of the endocrine glands, thus weakening our constitution. Correct, regular, rythmic breathing creates harmony within the body and the nervous system. We immediately feel relaxed and experience a sensation of physical and mental calm.

We shall be looking in detail at methods of breathing when we come to the topic on Pranayama exercises.

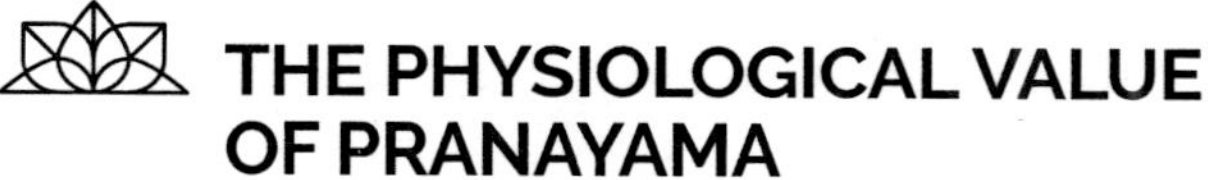

THE PHYSIOLOGICAL VALUE OF PRANAYAMA

Before going to Pranayama exercises, we shall examine how, and to what extent, Pranayama is able to affect the main systems of the body (nervous, endocrine, respiratory, circulatory and digestive) and how it ensures their harmonious and efficient functioning.

WHY DO WE BREATHE?

Two processes are absolutely essential to life: the absorption of oxygen by inhalation of air, and expulsion of carbonic gas through exhaling of air. We should bear in mind that the human body is constantly at work, even when it appears to be resting. All the body systems — circulatory, respiratory, digestive, endocrine and nervous — are constantly in operation. Such movement causes continous wear and tear of the body tissues involved. Losses have therefore to be repaired and made good, and waste-products evacuated. Nourishment must be supplied to repair such losses: it comes, not only from food and drink, but also from the air we breathe. Oxygen is the most important part of food. Life is impossible without it, even for a few minutes. When the blood reaches the lungs therefore, it draws the oxygen from the inhaled air and carries it to the various parts of the body through the circulatory system on returning to the lungs, the blood is full of carbonic gas collected from the tissues. It is the waste-product created by the body's mechanisms. If too much gas is allowed to remain in the body, it will become poisoned. It must therefore be evacuated by exhalation.

When veinous blood absorbs oxygen and evacuates carbon dioxide it is said to be arterialized. Veinous blood is first collected into the heart, then subsequently pumped into the lungs. Thence arterial blood is sent back to the heart to be distributed to the various parts of the body; it is once again brought back to the heart, this time as 'venous blood, and the process continues thus until the end of our lives.

If the quantity of carbon dioxide in the blood is above average, the respiratory centre becomes more active, i.e., we breathe faster. This can be very clearly seen when we exercise. In the opposite case, the respiratory system becomes calmer if the quantity of carbonic gas in the blood falls lower than normal, so that breathing slows down. One of the most important factors is the regulation of breath.

We shall now examine how Pranayama can help in the proper functioning of various systems within the body, beginning with the organs of evacuation: the kidneys and the bowels, which are situated in the abdomen. When breathing is normal, the alternate contraction and relaxing of the abdominal muscles, plus the rise and fall of the diaphragm, keep the kidneys and bowels moving, massaging them gently and continually. During Pranayama exercises, inhaling and exhaling, plus the holdings of the breath cause considerable movement and massage. Congestion is immediately removed due to the pressure exerted. The nerves and muscles controlling the kidney and intestinal movements are strengthened. They benefit not only from exercises during Pranayama but also for the remaining part of the day. This way the bowels and kidneys are rendered healthier due to Pranayama and can carry out their evacuatory functions more efficiently.

The same is true for the lungs. Healthy breathing depends on respiratory muscles and their elasticity. In Pranayama, the chest muscles are stretched to the maximum and the lungs opened as far as possible. They are thus better prepared to carry out their task.

Pranayama exercises are equally effective in the case of digestion and assimilation. The stomach, pancreas and liver all play a very important part in the digestive process and they too benefit from the various Pranayama exercises, and the massage given to them by the diaphragm and abdominal muscles. Many people with dyspepsia or constipation suffer from a liver which functions poorly or constantly gets congested. Pranayama exercises are excellent for relieving such congestion, stimulating a torpid pancreas and bringing improvement to all such gastric complaints. When the digestive system is functioning perfectly and correctly, the body receives a greater supply of the nutritious substances it needs.

It is essential that a living being absorb a certain quantity of oxygen to feed the blood. The quantity absorbed depends on the efficiency of the respiratory system. Insufficient breathing will reduce the absorption of oxygen into the blood and the tissues irrigated by blood lacking in oxygen will be under-nourished. Further, the intake of nutritious food will be quite useless unless the digestive system is working properly. Food will not get digested or suitably absorbed and much of it will be wasted. The body will receive only a small part of its nutritional content. It may be seen, therefore, that the respiratory and digestive systems must both work properly if the quality of the blood supplied to the body is to be maintained. More than any exercise, Pranayama can improve the supply of oxygen in the blood. It is during the practice of Pranayama that a large

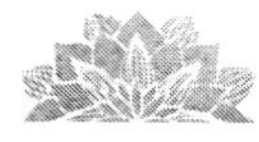

quantity of oxygen is absorbed, and proper functioning of the respiratory system maintained for the following twenty-four hours. The respiratory apparatus disciplined by these exercises improves breathing for the rest of the day, and much greater quantities of oxygen than normal are absorbed.

During the execution of the Pranayama Ujjayi (breathing that regenerates the endocrine glands), Bhastrika (the Bellows,) and Kapalabhati (breathing that revives the body), vibrations are created that spread to almost all the tissues of the organism, including the arteries, veins and capillary vessels. The heart, being the main organ of the circulation, becomes stronger. The whole circulatory system is toned up and ready to function properly.

Oxygen-rich and healthy blood and its distribution to all the nerves and glands ensures correct functioning of the nervous and endocrine systems. During Pranayama exercises, especially Bhastrika (the Bellows), the circulation becomes more efficient and the quality of the blood improves substantially. The supply of better quality blood feeds the endocrine glands, keeping them in good working order. It also reaches the cervical nerves — the network of nerves around the spinal column — and the sympathetic nerves. During *Puraka* (inhalation), the diaphragm is lowered and contracted, and the abdominal muscles are controlled, i.e., slightly contracted. The joint action of the diaphragm and abdominal muscles raises the lower part of the spinal column. During the practice of Jalandhara-Bandha or the Chin Lock the upper part of the spinal column is also raised. This action over the whole of the spine affects the sympathetic nerve and the roots of the nerves in the back.

In some ancient texts on Yoga, the nervous system is compared to a electricity generating plant and the network of wires carrying the current to the various factories and machines. The brain, spinal chord and sympathetic nerve constitute the power station, while the nerves leading away from the brain and spinal column represent the electric wires running through the factory, i.e., the human body.

All physical movement depends on impulses transmitted by the nerves from the brain to the muscles. If the power station is out of order, or there is a blockage in the current flowing down the electric wires, the machines will stop. Similarly, if the brain or nerves are damaged, or the latter are so worn that they no longer transmit impulses, physical movement stops. The digestion, circulation, and even breathing, are controlled by the brain and nerves following nervous impulses directed to the various organs responsible for these functions.

In the human body, the force of the current depends on the secretions of the endocrine glands. So, although the nervous system may be in complete working order, if the secretions of the endocrine glands are not available in sufficient quantity, or are not of the required quality, the force of nervous impulses, and even the nerves themselves, will be diminished. Consequently, physical movement will be lessened and the body will become sluggish. The nervous and endocrine systems are essential to human physiology, as are circulatory, the respiratory and digestive systems. The health of the nervous and endocrine system depends on these, and they are all exercised by Pranayama; the result is that the organism is healthier and full of vitality. All the great Yogis of India regarded Pranayama as the main exercise in the maintenance of the life-process and its perfect equilibrium.

THE PRACTICE OF PRANAYAMA

Let me start by earnestly entreating the reader to approach the practice of Pranayama with great care and under proper guidance.

Pranayama must be practised in a state of relaxation. If performed properly, there should never at any time be abrupt movements, violent inhalations or exhalations, nor should it provoke a feeling of suffocation.

Prana should be mastered very slowly and gradually, according to one's own capacities and physical limitations. The nasal cavities, membranes, throat, lungs, heart, nerves and diaphragm are the parts of the body actively involved. One should never hurry over Pranayama, for to do so is to play with one's own life. Any hypertension or incorrect practising may be harmful, especially to the nerves, heart, and lungs.

When practised correctly, Pranayama frees us from the majority of illnesses. We shall be assured of perfect health and peace of mind.

Air polluted by petrol fumes, and lack of sunshine due to the thick layer of smoke and haze hanging over cities, are responsible for the generally felt deficiency. The changes of temperature and climate affecting our body make it normal for the organism to feel totally exhausted at the end of each season of the year. We feel particularly tired and worn due to the build-up of toxins formed by each physical or intellectual effort made when atmospheric pressure is very low or when there are sudden changes in temperature; we seem to lack air and vital energy decreases, especially when the weather is sultry.

How can we combat this general build-up of toxins paralysing the muscles and nerves? How can the carbon dioxide that forms in the blood due to physical efforts be eliminated? Each Pranayama exercise shows us what to do — first, to clear the body completely, then to recharge it with healing oxygen that stimulates the circulation.

The ideal would of course be to get away from cities and go to the countryside to get some fresh air, from time to time. It is also recommended to carry out breathing exercises in a well-aired room with wide open windows, avoiding draughts, and wearing warm clothing if the weather is cold.

The best posture to practise Pranayama is the lotus position. If, for any reason, it is difficult to adopt, one can sit cross-legged or on one's heels. The important point is to keep the back, neck and head in a straight line from the base of the spinal column upwards, without feeling at all tired. There are also Pranayama exercises that can be executed standing up or lying on one's back.

To practise Pranayama properly, it is important, above all, to be the master of one's own rhythm. It is essential, therefore, to breathe regularly and according to a set rhythm. The Yogis measure time by counting their heartbeats. One can also use a watch.

HOW TO BREATHE PROPERLY

> 'Breath is life.'
>
> — *Veda*

To breathe is to live. Life is entirely dependent on the breath; all living things, including plants, must have air to live. Breath is ever-present, from the moment a baby fills its lungs, to the last gasp of a dying man. *'Life is nothing but a series of breaths,'* says a Hindu proverb.

While we may live without eating for several days, and without drinking for many hours, how many minutes can we last without breathing? Man must not only breathe to live, but should do so in such a way that he maintains constant vitality and avoids illness. Unfortunately, the number of people who know how to breathe properly is very small. Most people breathe in a very haphazard way as may be seen by cramped chests, stooping shoulders and the development of respiratory illnesses. It has been noted that unsatisfactory breathing habits decrease resilience and shorten life.

Whether they know it or not, some people breathe from the clavicle (the upper part of the chest), others from the thorax, and a third group from the diaphragm. Each one of these types of breathing is

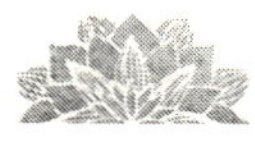

incomplete, for only one part of the lungs is filled with air. Research made in India by various Yoga institutes has shown that these kinds of breathing do not provide man with uniform development, whether physical, mental or spiritual.

The Yogis declare that the three types of breathing (from the diaphragm or abdomen, the thorax or median, clavicle or upper chest) should be combined, so that they form a single breathing pattern, similar to the movement of a wave. This is known as 'complete Yogic breathing'. It allows the lungs to be filled completely with oxygen, and is of the greatest value as it enables one to store a large amount of Prana. The Yogis also consider this type of breathing not only to ensure a long life by granting man unflagging vitality, and great powers of resistance, but also as an essential factor in his psychic and spiritual development.

The Yogis emphasize the point that complete Yogic breathing is the basis for all breathing exercises (Pranayama).

Complete Yogic breathing consists of three parts:
(1) the abdomen;
(2) the middle part of the chest (thorax);
(3) the upper part of the chest or collar bones (clavicle).

First, we shall examine each of the three types of breathing separately.

N.B. One should always inhale and exhale through the nose. The small screen of hair inside the nose not only filters the air, but also prevents impurities such as dust, harmful gases, minute insects, etc., from penetrating into the organism.

There is a Hindu saying: 'The nose is to breathe, the mouth is to eat and to speak whenever necessary.'

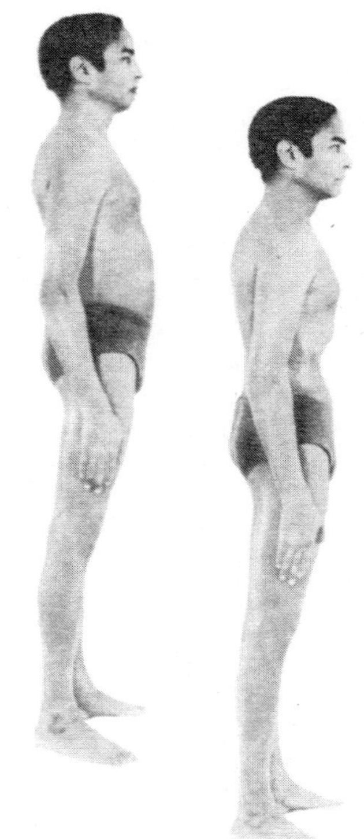

BREATHING FROM THE ABDOMEN

(Standing, sitting or lying on one's back)

The easiest method is to put the hands lightly on the abdomen so that its movements may be felt. During inhalation, the abdomen should be allowed to expand a little, like a bow, as the lower part of the lungs fills with air. During exhalation, the abdomen is allowed to sink in again. To be repeated several times.

THERAPEUTIC ADVANTAGES

This is an excellent internal massage for all the abdominal organs. It regularizes the functioning of the intestines and stimulates the digestion.

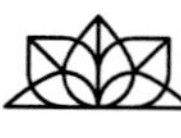

BREATHING FROM THE MIDDLE PART OF THE CHEST (THORAX)

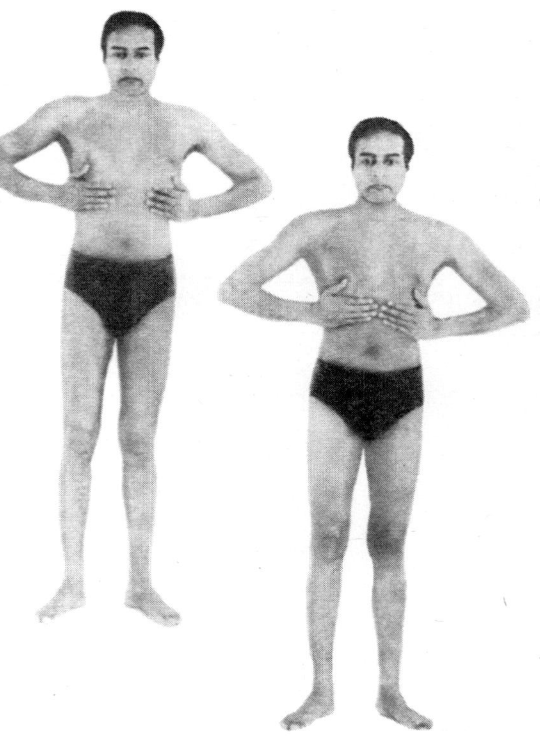

(Standing, sitting or lying on one's back)

Put the hands on either side of the ribs without pressing. Inhale slowly inflating the sides, then contract them by exhaling, like an accordian; repeat several times.

THERAPEUTIC ADVANTAGES

Purifies the blood, improves circulation and calms the heart.

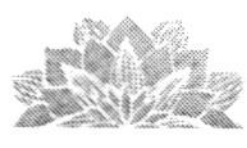

BREATHING FROM THE UPPER PART OF THE CHEST

(Standing, sitting or lying on one's back)

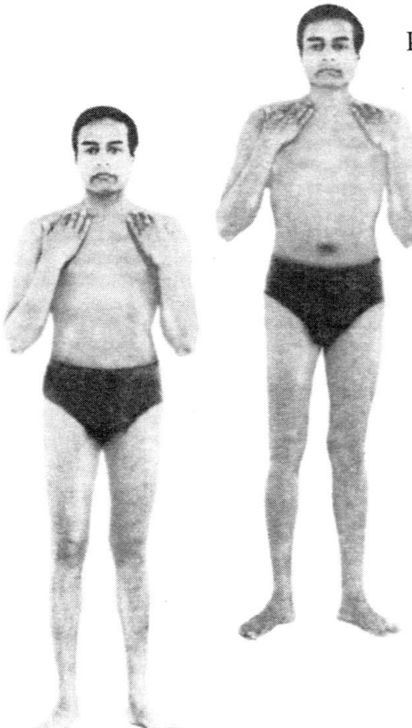

Put the hands on each side of the clavicle (upper chest) touching it with the fingers. Contract the stomach slightly. Inhale slowly pushing the clavicle upwards, then begin to exhale pushing it downwards. This exercise should also be repeated several times.

THERAPEUTIC ADVANTAGES

Thoroughly cleans and fortifies the upper chest.

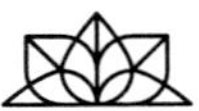

COMPLETE YOGIC BREATHING

(Standing, sitting or lying on the back)

In complete Yogic breathing, we combine abdominal, middle and upper parts of the chest in a wave-like movement. After exhaling completely we begin to inhale, letting the abdomen come out a little, and filling the lower part of the lungs, then expanding the ribs, whilst slightly drawing in the stomach until finally we fill the top part of the lungs.

In Sanskrit 'Puraka' means 'inhalation'.

Exhalation (Rechaka) begins with the abdomen being drawn in; then the ribs are contracted, and finally the collar bone lowered, thus completely emptying the lungs.

The whole process of inhaling and exhaling should be done as one smooth, continuous movement, like a wave, and the volume of breath while inhaling should be the same.

To begin with, it is quite difficult to breathe with this gentle, continuous movement; once the habit has been acquired, however, this wave-like breathing will come almost naturally. With a little patience and perseverance the desired results will be achieved.

THERAPEUTIC ADVANTAGES

There are so many benefits from complete Yogic breathing that they almost require a separate book to themselves. Complete Yogic breathing is of importance to all those men, women or children who wish to enjoy good health.

We should bear in mind that exercise of the external muscles is not all that is required: the internal organs also need exercise, and this is why complete Yogic breathing should be regarded as a gift.

Let us take, for example, the role of the diaphragm. Every movement of the respiratory organs makes those of nutrition and digestion vibrate, whilst supplying a larger quantity of blood to invigorate and massage various organs. If they are not treated in this way, they will remain sluggish and refuse to function properly: deficient movement of the diaphragm is the cause of many illnesses.

Complete Yogic breathing brings all of the respiratory organs into play, guards against pulmonary infections in general, and is very important in preventing asthma and heart trouble. It helps in maintaining the individual's perfect health. It can, revive the body when completely exhausted, or calms both mind and nervous system.

Similarly, Yogic breathing exercises are intended to help accumulate Prana. It is possible, not only to increase the quantity of Prana absorbed by deep and regular inhalation, but also to consciously direct it by exhalation to all parts of the body, so animating the latter; a much greater supply of oxygen is thus brought into the bloodstream. This way the vital organs, endocrine glands, nervous centres and body tissues are better nourished.

Remarkable results have been obtained at the Institute of Yoga Research, Lonavla, especially in the field of cardiac and high blood-pressure.

Abundant absorption of Prana calms the nervous system. Heartbeats become regular and the lungs are thoroughly aired. We are filled with a feeling of mental and physical peace.

RHYTHMIC BREATHING

This Pranayama is neither difficult nor dangerous, so everyone can practise it. Rhythmic breathing has two variations:

— during the first, inhalation takes exactly the same time as exhalation.

— during the second, the two take the same amount of time, but there is a pause between inhalation and exhalation equal to half of the time they each take.

For this type of breathing, it is important to concentrate mentally on the rhythm before becoming used to it.

Yogis time their breathing rhythm taking into account the rate of their heartbeat which may differ from person to person. The important point is to adjust the breathing to one's own rhythm. This should only be done after a minute of relaxation. To count the heartbeats and establish a suitable breathing rhythm, the pulse should be taken while counting from 1 to 6. This should be repeated until the rhythm is clear in one's mind. By practising this type of breathing, one can achieve equilibrium of the nervous system.

TECHNIQUE

When performing the first variation of the breathing pattern, sit cross-legged holding the chest, neck and head in a straight vertical line, with hands on knees (those who find it difficult to sit cross-legged may perform this exercise lying on their back). Inhale as in complete Yogic breathing, mentally counting 6 heartbeats, then slowly exhale through the nostrils, again counting to 6. Repeat the exercise several times.

For the second variation the posture is the same. Inhale deeply and count from 1 to 6, hold the breath and count from 1 to 3, now exhale slowly counting from 1 to 6 again. Stop breathing to a count of 3, then start to inhale again, etc.

It is imperative to have proper guidance as to the number and duration of exercises.

The beginner should concentrate particularly on acquiring a rhythmic breathing pattern without straining to prolong the duration of inhalation and exhalation. Only after long practice will he be able to count up to 16 beats instead of 6. By practising this type of breathing, one is eventually able to communicate soothing rhythmic vibrations to the whole of the body.

Once rhythmic breathing has become almost automatic, we ought to feel that each inhalation is filling us with calm, and each exhalation transmitting it to the tiniest fibres of the body, like a current passing through our cells. We should consciously absorb this wave of calm with each breath taken. We shall find that the whole body becomes rhythmical and harmonious, hence, due to

rhythmic breathing all the molecules in the body tend to move in the same direction.

THERAPEUTIC ADVANTAGES

A totally exhausted body revives and the most tired frayed nerves become calm. We experience genuine rest, better even than that of sleep, because it is acquired. consciously. A relaxed expression appears on the face, wrinkles soften, as do the features. We sleep better and a new life flows through the body.

Rhythmic breathing brings health to body and mind. It allows more oxygen into the body, relieves the ageing of muscles, helps to re-establish the equilibrium of the nervous and neuro-vegetal systems. It also eliminates anxiety by acting on the sympathetic nerve and the thalamus (interior region of the brain).

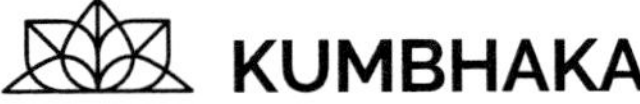

KUMBHAKA

(Retention of the breath)

PRECAUTIONS

While the breath is being held, one should not experience any feeling of suffocation. Once the exercise is over, it should be possible to breathe normally without the slightest effort. The average person should not, generally speaking, hold his breath longer than thirty-two seconds, unless the exercise is done under the supervision of a Yoga expert. Those suffering from illnesses affecting the heart or lungs should refrain from performing this exercise.

TECHNIQUE

Sitting cross-legged or in the lotus position, one inhales as in complete Yogic breathing, then holds the breath for six seconds initially. One can then add one second each day until the maximum of thirty-two seconds is reached. One then exhales, following the same rhythm as for inhaling.

THERAPEUTIC ADVANTAGES

Yoga experience has shown that the holding of the breath for a certain length of time, according to individual capacity, has beneficial effects on the organism. The practice of Pranayama, including the holding of the breath, allows large quantities of oxygen and Prana to be stored. It also acts effectively on the respiratory organs, digestion, circulation and nervous system.

Control of the breathing allows us on the one hand to absorb more oxygen and Prana, and on the other, by re-establishing the equilibrium of our positive and negative energies, to bring our mental and physical states into perfect harmony.

With regular practice of complete Yogic breathing one not only avoids problems affecting the lungs, liver, gall-bladder, stomach and heart, but also maintains good health and vital forces; this also accounts for the development of the will-power.

ANULOMA VILOMA OR NADI SHODHANA PRANAYAMA

(Alternate breathing)

In Sanskrit, 'Nadi' signifies a 'channel' allowing the passage of vital energy of Prana. According to Yoga, inhaling by the right nostril produces heat in the body, and inhaling by the left produces cold. This is why the Yogis call the right nostril Surya Nadi (sun nostril) and the left Chandra Nadi (moon nostril).

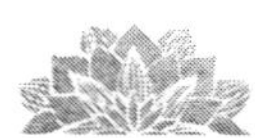

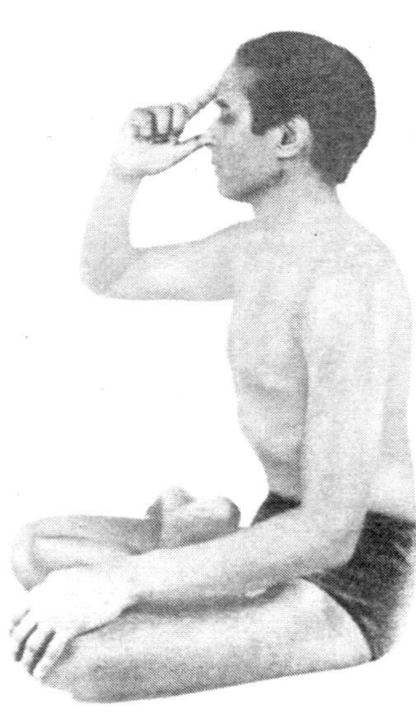

PRECAUTIONS

This Pranayama must be carried out very carefully, and to begin with, the full cycle should not be repeated more than three times.

Those suffering from cardiac complaints or high blood pressure, or those with weak lungs, should at no time practise this exercise to include the holding of the breath (Kumbhaka) without proper guidance.

TECHNIQUE

Sitting in the Padmasana position or cross-legged, place the index finger of the right hand in the centre of the forehead between the eyebrows. One should begin by exhaling completely; then close the right nostril with the thumb and inhale through the left nostril counting four seconds, hold to a count of sixteen, then open the right nostril while closing the left with middle finger. Exhale through the right nostril to a count of eight heartbeats. Keeping the fingers in the same position, inhale through the right nostril counting four beats, then hold the breath to a count of sixteen before exhaling through the left nostril counting up to eight heartbeats. This forms the complete cycle.

To begin with, it is always better to follow the set rhythm 1:2:2 for this exercise which includes inhalation, retention of the breath and exhalation. After long practice (2 or 3 months minimum) one may proceed to 1:4:2.

THERAPEUTIC ADVANTAGES

This is one of the most important Pranayamas for establishing the equilibrium of the positive and negative currents bringing life to the body. It calms and purifies nerves, stabilizes mind and increases mental faculties. It helps cure certain types of headache.

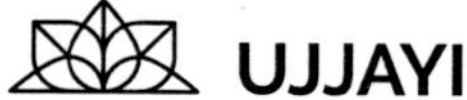

UJJAYI

(Energy-renewing Pranayama)

The distinctive feature of this Pranayama is that the glottis is half-closed, producing a low continuous sound throughout the breathing exercise.

PRECAUTIONS

Neither the facial muscles nor those of the nose should be contracted. The exercise is often practised without the breath being held. Exhalation is twice as long as inhalation, i.e., 1:2. When practising Ujjayi to include holding of the breath, the rhythm is 1:2:2 (e.g. inhalation 4 seconds, retention 8, exhalation 8).

TECHNIQUE

The Padmasana, Siddhasana or cross-legged position is adopted (the exercise may also be performed standing). Once the breath contained in the lungs has been completely exhaled, the glottis is partially closed and air inhaled through both nostrils, while expanding the thoracic cage. The abdominal muscles must be kept under control and contracted slightly throughout inhalation. The air should then be exhaled while the glottis is kept half-closed and the abdominal muscles contracted tighter and tighter, until the lungs are completely empty and the thoracic cage sunk inwards.

To begin with, this exercise should only be repeated three times; later on two extra repetitions may be added each week to reach a total of 15 (without the breath being held).

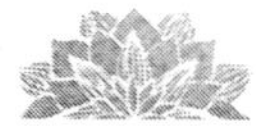

While practising this Ujjayi to improve the physical state, one should concentrate at each inhalation on the energy-renewing breath and, at each exhalation, on the absorption of energy.

When performing the exercise with a spiritual end in view, one should imagine that with each breath taken, a divine current passes through the body.

THERAPEUTIC ADVANTAGES

Digestive and pulmonary complications (e.g., indigestion, coughing, etc.) may be avoided by the practice of this exercise. When performed daily, Ujjayi has both preventive and curative influence. By increasing the vitality, it strengthens both the circulatory and the nervous system.

Low blood pressure is raised to a normal level, the endocrine glands (especially the thyroid) are greatly stimulated.

When practised under supervision, the exercise is ideal for those suffering from high blood pressure and coronary disorders.

KAPALABHATI

(Breathing that revitalizes the body)

In Sanskrit, *Kapala* means 'skull' and *Bhati* 'to shine'. It is one of the six purification exercises known to Hatha Yoga. The object is to purify the channels inside the nose in addition to all the other parts of the respiratory system, thus allowing the brain to be cleared as well.

PRECAUTIONS

Those in good health may perform this exercise, but those suffering from pulmonary or cardiac disorders should only undertake it under the guidance of experienced teachers of Yoga. All those who practise it should, in any case, stop at the slightest sign of fatigue.

TECHNIQUE

Kapalabhati is a respiratory exercise for the abdomen and diaphragm (to be performed sitting either in the lotus position or simply cross-legged, with hands on knees).

In other exercises the accent has been on inhalation, retention and exhalation; but here, in Kapalabhati, it is solely on exhalation. It is the only exercise that does not require deep breathing.

Once the thoracic cage has been expanded, it does not move, only the diaphragm and abdominal muscles do.

The air filling the thoracic cage is expelled without pause in continuous, rapid exhalations.

One should start with 5 to 7 such exhalations, but these may subsequently be increased, according to the individual's capacity.

THERAPEUTIC ADVANTAGES

This exercise enables us to eliminate a large quantity of the toxins contained in the body, by filling the blood with oxygen and purifying the tissues and nerves.

This Pranayama clears the nasal cavities and lungs. It is a remedy against deficiencies in the lymphatic system, and mucus in the nose and lungs. The exercise brings relief from asthma and tones

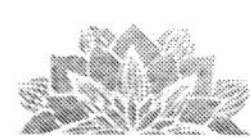

up the body. It fortifies the salivary glands and expels bacteria that have penetrated into the nose. The solar plexus is recharged with vital energy, the circulation and digestive system function more efficiently. The exercise also helps develop the powers of concentration.

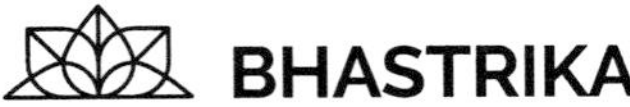 BHASTRIKA

(Bellows)

In Sanskrit, *Bhastrika* means 'bellows'. This exercise is characterized by continual exhalation of breath, producing a sound similar to a blacksmith's bellows. In fact, it is nothing more than a combination of Kapalabhati and Ujjayi. It begins with Kapalabhati, ends with Ujjayi, includes holding of the breath.

PRECAUTIONS

This type of Pranayama must be practised with great care; one should stop at the slightest sign of fatigue, for the body will become exhausted very quickly if the exercise is overdone. Those with a fragile constitution suffering from high or low blood pressure should not attempt this kind of exercise.

TECHNIQUE

One sits cross-legged or in the lotus position. Air is expelled in quick successive exhalations through the nose. After a certain number of such exhalations (according to the individual's capacity), a deep breath is taken half closing the glottis. The air is then held by closing the glottis completely. The nostrils should also be blocked with the thumb, ring finger and little finger of the right hand while the head is lowered and the chin firmly buried in the hollow above the sternum (Jalandhar Bandha or Chin-Lock). The air is then expelled with the glottis half-open. The rhythm is 1:2:2, making one complete Bhastrika exercise. One should start by performing it twice, then gradually increase the number of times as indicated by the Yoga instructor.

Variation: The second part of this exercise may also be done without half-closing the glottis.

THERAPEUTIC ADVANTAGES

This Pranayama spreads warmth all over the body and has a purifying effect. It regenerates the liver, spleen, pancreas and fortifies the abdominal muscles. The digestion improves and one experiences a general feeling of well-being.

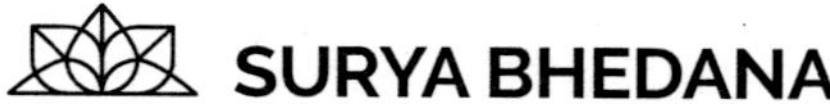

SURYA BHEDANA

(Breathing that revitalizes the nervous system)

Surya means 'sun' and *Bhedana* 'to open or unfold oneself'. In this Pranayama, one inhales through the right nostril and exhales by the left.

PRECAUTIONS

Those suffering from cardiac complaints, or have weak lungs, should not hold the breath. If this Pranayama is practised to include the retention of the breath however, those suffering from high blood pressure will extract the maximum benefit from it — providing they practise it under proper guidance.

TECHNIQUE

One should sit either cross-legged, or in the Padmasana or Siddhasana position. Air is inhaled through the right nostril and the

breath held until pressure to exhale is felt. Once the breath has been held in accordance with personal capacity, it is exhaled by the left nostril, but the process is much slower than inhalation.

It should be noted at this point that, to begin with, the practice of holding the breath should be gradually developed according to individual capacity. Impatience or over hastiness during this exercise may damage the lungs and even be the cause of an incurable illness. The rhythm of inhalation, retention and exhalation should be 1:2:2, at the beginning. Only after long practice should the following rhythm be adopted — 1:4:2. To begin with, this exercise should only be repeated 5 times, working up to 7.

THERAPEUTIC ADVANTAGES

This Pranayama brings the body temperature into equilibrium and controls the functions of the catabolism. The powers of digestion are increased and the nervous system fortified. The sinuses are also cleared.

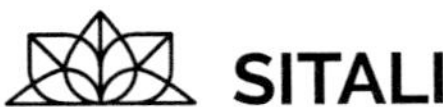

SITALI

(Breathing that refreshes)

The name of this Pranayama is derived from the refreshing effect it has on the body. In this the air is breathed in through the mouth and not the nose.

PRECAUTIONS

Those suffering from high blood pressure should omit the holding of the breath. Those with cardiac complaints should not do this Pranayama.

TECHNIQUE

The position to be adopted is Padmasana, Siddhasana, or simply cross-legged. The tongue is drawn out of the mouth roughly one inch. Its sides are turned upwards (lengthwise) like a freshly rolled leaf. We inhale by drawing in the air through the channel formed by the tongue making an 'SSSSS' sound until the lungs are completely filled. Once inhalation has been accomplished, the tongue is drawn in, the lips closed and the breath held for 5 to 10 seconds. The air is then let out slowly through the nose. This completes the cycle. The exercise should be repeated two or three times, followed by complete relaxation. The number of cycles should gradually be increased.

THERAPEUTIC ADVANTAGES

This Pranayama refreshes and tones up the body, activating the liver and bile, with beneficial effects on the circulation and body temperature.

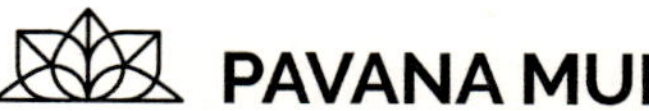

PAVANA MUKTASANA

(Relieving gas contained in the body)

In Sanskrit *Pavana* means 'wind' and *Mukta* 'to rid oneself of something'. This posture enables the body to be freed of the gas it contains.

TECHNIQUE

Lie on the back with the legs folded against the chest. Wrap the arms tightly around the knees and breathe deeply (as in complete Yogic breathing). Breathe out slowly and fully through the nostrils while pressing the knees closely on the abdomen. When breathing

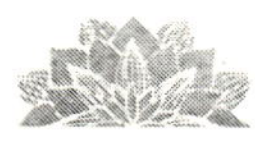

in, relax the pressure from the arms. Repeat the exercise several times.

THERAPEUTIC ADVANTAGES

All the gas that tends to accumulate in the organism is expelled.

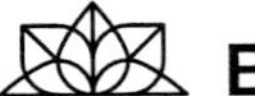

BREATHING THAT PURIFIES

PRECAUTIONS

Those with high blood pressure, cardiac complaints, or weak lungs should avoid practising this exercise.

TECHNIQUE

One stands with the legs slightly apart. A slow, deep breath is taken through the nose as in complete Yogic breathing. Having held the breath for several seconds, the lips are pressed against the teeth, leaving a small, narrow opening. The air contained in the lungs is forced out through the opening in a number of small exhalations until the lungs are completely empty. It is important to remember that the air must be forced out through the narrow opening with a great deal of effort, otherwise this Pranayama will not produce any beneficial effect. This exercise may be repeated several times according to the individual's capacity, but without tiring the lungs.

BREATHING THAT FORTIFIES THE NERVES

TECHNIQUE

Stand with the legs slightly apart and having exhaled, breathe in slowly as in complete Yogic breathing. Now raise the arms horizontally in front with palms facing upwards and gently raise them to the level of the shoulders. Hold the breath, close the hands and clench the fists while contracting the muscles of the arms. Bring the fists in briskly towards the body and then push them out slowly as before. Repeat the movement several times, but avoid becoming tired. Now exhale slowly through the nose and lean forward to relax the muscles of the arms completely, letting them hang down loosely.

THERAPEUTIC ADVANTAGES

This exercise is held to be one of the most powerful stimulants of the nerves. It develops the energy and vitality because it causes a large quantity of Prana to be distributed throughout the body. The mental faculties are increased and one gains self-confidence.

N.B. This exercise is not recommended for those with a weak heart or lungs.

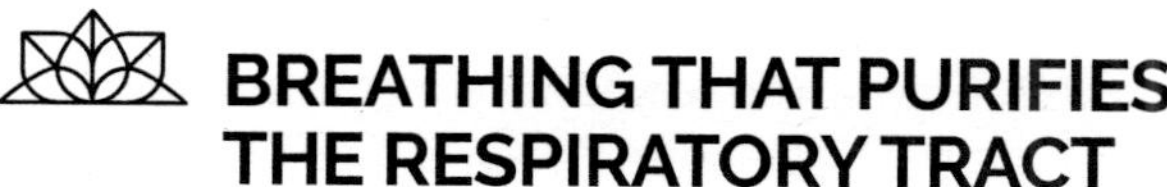

BREATHING THAT PURIFIES THE RESPIRATORY TRACT

TECHNIQUE

This exercise may be performed standing with the legs slightly apart. Inhale slowly as in complete Yogic breathing while raising the arms vertically. Having held the breath for a few seconds, lean forward rapidly allowing the arms to hang down loosely while exhaling forcefully through the mouth. This will produce a

'HHHHH ...' sound coming from the air suddenly expelled from the lungs. Raise your body up slowly, raising the arms above the head and breathing in deeply through the nose. Then exhale, again through the nose, while lowering arms. Relax completely. Repeat the exercise several times.

THERAPEUTIC ADVANTAGES

The circulation is enlivened, the lungs fully cleared, and the body experiences a feeling of warmth. This exercise helps us maintain a healthy mind and resist outside influences. It also gets rid of depression.

VARIATION

TECHNIQUE

One can also lie on one's back and inhale deeply and slowly, as in complete Yogic breathing, while stretching out the arms behind the head. The breath is held for several seconds and then suddenly one brings up the knees and presses them against the abdomen wrapping the arms tightly around them. The breath is exhaled through the mouth at the same time. After a few seconds, one breathes in slowly and deeply through the nose lifting the arms behind the head and stretching out the legs on the ground again. Then the arms are lowered while the breath is exhaled from the lungs through the nose. The exercise may be repeated several times before one relaxes completely.

THERAPEUTIC ADVANTAGES

The same as for standing.

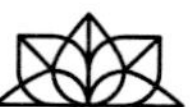

HOW TO REVITALIZE THE WHOLE BODY

TECHNIQUE

This is performed lying on the back, the position in which we feel completely at ease and relaxed (as in shavasana). We breathe slowly and deeply as in complete Yogic breathing. We should constantly bear in mind that each time we inhale we are absorbing Prana and when we exhale, we send it throughout the body to its tiniest fibres. It is suggested that one stay in this position for five to ten minutes, while continuing to breathe in the same manner.

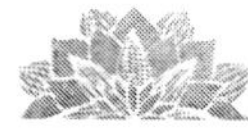

3

The Asanas (Yogic Postures)

THE PHYSIOLOGICAL FUNCTIONS OF THE HUMAN BODY AND THE ASANAS

According to ancient Hindu tradition, god Shiva is said to have demonstrated 8,400,000 Asanas — as many as there are living species — to enable man to keep his body in perfect health, so that he could attain the highest level of his spiritual development.

Experiments were carried out on a number of Asanas by the ancient great Yogis, who revealed them in order to help man.

In ancient Sanskrit texts such as the *Shiva Samhita* (chapter III, verses 84-91), 84 postures are mentioned, while in the *Gheranda Samhita* (the second *Upadesha*) only 32 are described. In fact, however, a mere 20-25 are required to maintain or re-establish perfect health. Experience has shown me that the effects of the *Asanas* (yogic postures), *Pranayama* (control and regularization of the breath), *Mudras* (endurance exercises) and *Bandhas* (contraction exercises) are all extremely beneficial to the well-being of the human beings.

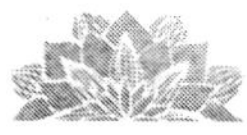

No method of physical exercises, no sport, can supply the human body with benefits equal to those offered by Yogic postures, without at the same time tiring or exhausting it. The role they play in the protection of vital energy and the maintenance of good health is quite remarkable. Not only do they give the entire body an external massage, but also provide absolutely unique exercises of the internal organs.

Health depends on the state of the tissues and the cells composing them. Muscles can only preserve their force and elasticity if they are regularly stretched and contracted.

Before dealing with the practical aspects of the Asanas, we shall first look at the various physiological functions of the body. The appropriate Asanas indicated here are able to maintain these functious perfectly and provide the whole body with better organic force. If we are to animate, regenerate, strengthen and develop the body both consciously and at will, we should be familiar, not only with the head, trunk, legs and arms, but also the internal organs, going from the smallest unit of cells to the whole of the muscular system.

The body is composed of cells. A cell represents the smallest organic unit in the body. It is composed of protoplasm, considered to be the physical basis of life, without which there can be no living thing. Protoplasm enables the cell to become an independent organic unit, helping it to survive, nourish itself and grow individually, even to reproduce. Such cells vary in shape, according to the structure of the organs to which they belong. As they are always active they should be nourished by proteins, fats, sugar, salts, water and oxygen, so that they are able to produce the protoplasm that enables them to live and function properly.

Tissues are formed from a combination of several cells. All organs in the body are made of tissue. Each organ has its own form and function. When the muscles contract, each muscular tissue contracts with them. The glands secretes various juices when active. Nerve tissues also transmit impulses when functioning properly.

In order to keep tissues in perfect health, they should be nourished well and regularly. The endocrine glands should be properly maintained to keep them in perfect condition; this is to eliminate waste products so that the nervous system may function correctly.

It is known that tissue feeds on various proteins, fats, sugars, salts as well as oxygen, all brought to them by the blood. Such food depends not only on the quality and quantity of what we eat or drink, but also on our digestive powers and the way nourishment is assimilated. For tissues to be properly nourished, both the circulation and the digestive system have to function properly.

The main organs of the digestive system are stomach, small intestine, pancreas and liver situated in the abdomen. Throughout the 24 hours that we breathe in and out, these organs are gently massaged by abdominal wall which pushes them rhythmically inwards and upwards. Such automatic massage is very efficient when the muscles in the abdomen are strong and flexible. If they are weak, however, the result is indigestion and many other abdominal disorders. To help the muscles maintain their force and elasticity, therefore, we must practise postures designed to stretch and contract them. During the practice of Salabhasana (the Grasshopper position), the Bhujangasana (the Cobra position), and the Dhanurasana (the Bow position), we stretch the abdominal muscles whilst at the same time contracting the muscles in the back. When we perform the Halasana (the Plough position), Yoga-Mudra (the Symbol of Yoga), and Paschimottanasana (stretching of the back and leg muscles), we have to do the opposite, i.e., tightly contract the abdominal muscles to their fullest extent while stretching those of the back. We contract and stretch the abdominal muscles that pass from one side to the other in the same way by practising the Ardha-Matsyendrasana (simplified Matsyendra position) and the Vakrasana (twisting of the spinal column). The

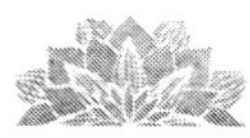

vertical massage of the abdominal organs may be obtained by the practice of the Uddiyana-Bandha (raising of the diaphragm).

All the Asanas indicated above not only preserve the solidity and elasticity of the abdominal muscles ensuring proper digestion and assimilation. It is in this way that the digestive system distributes proteins, fats, sugar and salt equally throughout the body.

The other important system nourishing the tissues is the circulatory system. Blood is pumped in the body by the heart, passing through the arteries, veins and capillaries. The heart is the most important organ because its contraction and relaxation push the blood through the body.

Uddiyana-Bandha gives the heart an excellent massage by raising the diaphragm. The increase and decrease of pressure on the cavity helps maintain the cardiac muscle in good health. Viparitakarani (inverted posture), Sarvangasana (head-stand) and Halasana (the plough posture) alternately augment and diminish pressure on the heart. The same is true of Salabhasana (the Grasshopper position), Bhujangasana (the Cobra position) and Dhanurasana (Bow position). Such alternate pressures maintain the correct functioning of the heart. The veins, helped by the arteries and capillaries, carry blood to the heart, struggling in places against the force of gravity.

Three inversion postures, Viparitakarani, Sarvangasana and Sirshasana are excellent for keeping the veins healthy. In the inverted posture, the veins in the lower part of the body are relieved of the strenuous effort they usually have to make to carry the blood back to the heart, so that it flows without difficulty. Not only does this help the veins maintain their health, but also strengthens the muscles of the heart. In this way the circulatory system carries the blood in correct proportion required by all the tissues of the body.

OXYGEN

Oxygen, like the other four substances (protein, fat, sugar and salt), is brought to the tissues by the blood (haemoglobin). Unlike the other foodstuffs, however, it does not enter the bloodstream through the digestive system, but through the respiratory system.

We can only breathe correctly and absorb the oxygen we need if our lungs are strong and in good working order. Not unless all the air-cells of the lungs take an active part in the breathing process can we be certain that they are in good health. Salabhasana is highly beneficial to the activity of these cells and the elasticity of the lungs. By holding the breath, even for a few seconds, the air is forced to enter each pulmonary cell, thus inflating it and making it more active. It is helpful in preserving the elasticity of the lung tissue. In addition to Salabhasana and Uddiyana-Bandha also helps to strengthen respiratory muscles by deep inhalation and exhalation.

Viparitakarani, Sarvangasana and Matsyasana keep the respiratory tract clear, so that the oxygen absorbed by the lungs is supplied in the required quantity to the tissues.

THE ENDOCRINE GLANDS

The health of tissues does not only depend on the sufficient supply of protein, fats, salts and oxygen, but also on the internal secretions of the endocrine glands.The most important of these are the pituitary, pineal gland, thyroid, parathyroid, adrenal glands and the gonads or sexual glands.

They are called endocrine glands or ductless glands because their secretions are internal and pass directly into the bloodstream, without flowing through channels of their own. Hence the endocrine glands have no ducts, that is why they are also called 'ductless'. An insufficient secretion from anyone of them could entail serious consequences.

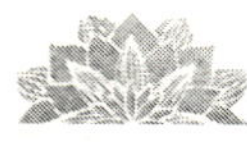

The *pituitary* for example, which is situated inside the skull just behind the nose, below the brain is the master gland affecting all the others, including the sexual glands. If one eats too many fats and carbohydrates over a number of years, the glands tend to weaken, and the effect on pituitary can be detrimental. This will result in excess fat deposits around the chest and abdomen.

The *pineal gland* is also situated inside the skull, at the base of the brain. It is the seat of the highest faculties, such as occult powers: clairvoyance, telepathy, and so on. It plays an important part in preserving the equilibrium of the endocrine system. Practice of Sirshasana (head-stand) is the best way of keeping the pineal and pituitary glands in perfect health. If for some reason it is not possible to practise Sirshasana, the same benefit may mostly be obtained by Viparitakarani, Saravangasana and Matsyasana.

The *thyroid glands* lie in the front or foreground of the throat, and *parathyroid glands* are located at each side of the thyroid.The thyroid is one of nature's strongest agents protecting the human body; it has been called a 'watchman' standing between the physical and mental body. Hormones are secreted by this gland that are essential in keeping the body alert. The thyroid gland regulates metabolism. One of the thyroid's tasks is to burn fats, but in case of malfunction or hypothyroidism, fat deposits may build up. Mental sluggishness, loss of memory, lack of awareness of time, constant desire for sleep, and depression are the symptoms of thyroid insufficiency. When this gland overworks, i.e., in case of hyper-thyroid, the situation is reversed. Excessive weight-loss, tension, insomnia, palpitations, nervousness, agitation and continual haste are the symptoms of hyperthyroid complaints. Thyroid degeneration is the cause of many illnesses, e.g., accelerated ageing and even premature death, while malfunctioning of the parathyroid glands may cause strange allergies, painful cramps and spasms. We may preserve the correct equilibrium of the thyroid and parathyroid — even to a great age — by regular practice of Viparitakarani, Sarvangasana and Matsyasana.

The *adrenal glands* are located like small caps on the top of each kidney. They secrete the hormone adrenaline which flows into the blood arousing the body's defenses; they warn us to be ready for action, and help us in difficult situations. In perfect condition, they make us feel energetic and active. Should they be in bad health, they raise the blood pressure and are the cause of many other disorders affecting the circulation. Bhujangasana, Uddiyana-Bandha and Dhanurasana keep the adrenal glands in perfect condition.

The *Gonads* or *sexual glands* are the testicles for a man and the ovaries for a woman. They are situated in the pelvic area. They produde both internal and external secretions. The latter are the origin of reproduction, while the former revivify the whole of the body. Sarvangasana and Uddiyana have proved to be highly effective in maintaining the testicles and ovaries in perfect health.

The fact that the various vegetatvie functions are in good condition mainly depends on the endocrine glands. If these are disturbed, they may provoke serious complaints.

Hence we may conclude that the practice of Asanas is able to ensure the health of the endocrine glands, so that they may produce the secretions required by the tissues.

To keep the tissues healthy: *the complete elimination of the body's waste-products is required.*

The uric acid contained in urine, urea, bile and other faecal substances are waste-products that gives rise to various ailments if not removed promptly. We can eliminate them only when the digestive, respiratory and urinary systems are functioning properly. They may be kept in good order by the practice of Dhanurasana, Bhujangasana and Uddiyana which are beneficial to the kidneys.

For proper maintenance of the tissues it is necessary the nervous system should function properly. The most important part of our

nervous system is the brain. The network of nerves starts from the brain, passes along the spinal chord whence it diverges into the whole of the body. If the nerve-connections are frayed or broken, the tissues are no longer able to carry out their function properly — with catastrophic results for the body. If the nerve-connections are in good health, the tissues will also be active and healthy.

Sirshasana and Viparitakarani are excellent for ensuring the proper functioning of the brain and cranial nerves, for these postures supply them with a rich influx of blood. All the other Yoga postures designed to stretch the body forwards, backwards, from one side to the other and twist to the right, then the left, maintain the tissues perfectly elastic and keep the spinal column healthy. Uddiyana-Bandha is particulary salutary for the spinal column and the sympathetic nerves.

In this way Yoga postures are able to maintain the whole nervous system in good health.

We have now seen how the constant supply of suitable foodstuffs, the regular secretions of the endocrine glands, the complete elimination of waste products, and the proper functioning of the nervous system all help keep the tissues healthy by the practice of Asanas.

Good health depends not only on the physical activities of the individual, but also on the *muscles in his body*. If we have no muscles, or they are unhealthy, it is absolutely impossible to carry out physical labour properly: we simply do not have the strength. Asanas are able to maintain and improve our muscle-power. In the following section, we shall examine the Asanas by giving a complete and practical description of them.

THE PRACTICE OF THE ASANAS

One should constantly bear in mind that the body must never be forced nor fatigued during the execution of postures. The moment we feel the slightest pain, we should take it as a sign that it is time to stop. Each posture should be performed slowly, carefully, gradually and patiently. One should not go too fast. For older people, postures may be simplified according to individual needs. Asanas should be practised on an empty stomach. Unless the above advice is followed, the results will not be positive.

If the exercises are not performed as they should be or as advised, one will begin to feel uncomfortable and unwell after a few days. This is the sign that something is wrong with the way Yoga is being practised.

When the postures are correctly and properly done, however, they produce a feeling of lightness and well-being that is both physical and mental; one has the impression of a freshness that induces a state of total relaxation.

PADMASANA

The Lotus Position

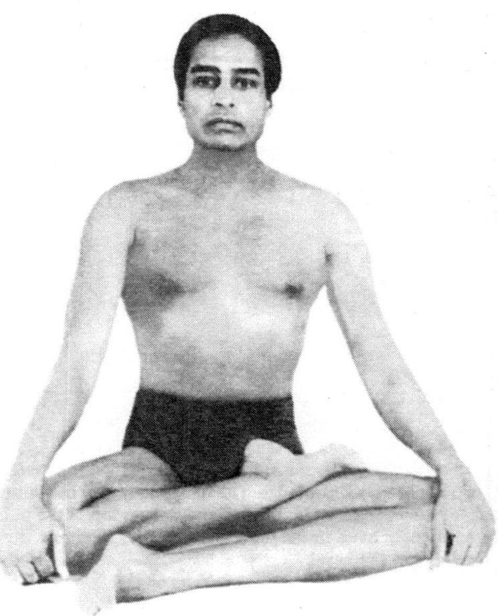

TECHNIQUE

Padmasana is a meditation posture. Those suffering from stiff legs, knees, ankles, etc., can overcome this difficulty by regular practice combined with patience and perseverance.

We begin by placing the right foot on the left thigh and the left foot on the right thigh. The position of heels is adjusted so that they are

both pressing on the nearest part of the abdomen. The hands are kept open and rest on the knees, palms in the air with the tips of the index finger touching the thumb, thus forming a small circle called 'Jnana Mudra'. The index finger represents the individual soul and the thumb the universal one. The union of the two symbolizes Knowledge. The hands may also rest flat on the knees. Another position for the hands is to place them one on top of the other, palms in the air, with the back of the right hand inside the left hand. They then rest quite naturally in the pit of the stomach below the navel.

It is important to keep the head and spinal column straight, but without straining.

THERAPEUTIC ADVANTAGES

This posture develops physical and mental stability, calms the nerves, relieves the stiffness of knees and joints, and guards against rheumatism. The abdominal region receives a copious supply of blood from the point where the abdominal aorta divides. The effect of this is to invigorate the coccyx region and the nerves of the sacrum. The entire body is kept in complete equilibrium.

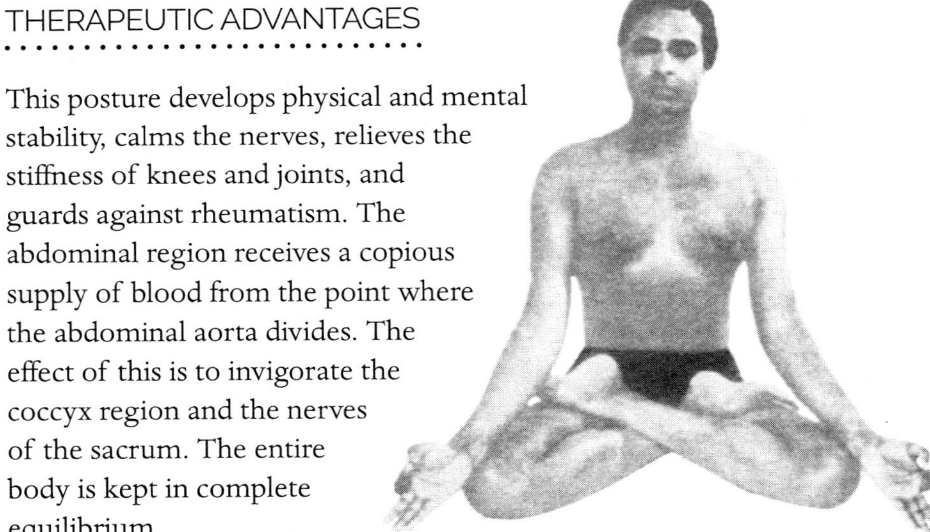

N.B.: The following meditation postures, such as Siddhasana, Svastika and Samasana all have same therapeutic effects.

SIDDHASANA

Posture of the Adept

TECHNIQUE

Care must be taken not to hurt the genitals; the spinal column should remain vertical. To avoid unpleasant pressure, the time spent on the daily practice of this exercise should be increased gradually.

The heel of the left foot is placed against the perineum, and the right foot is brought up to the pubic bone just above the genital organs. These should be carefully placed under the right heel in such a way that there is no pressure bearing on them. The hands may be held in the Jnana Mudra position, placed one on top of the other, or quite simply allowed to rest flat on the knees as in Padmasana.

THERAPEUTIC ADVANTAGES

This posture develops physical and mental stability, calms the nerves, relieves stiffness in the knees and joints and prevents rheumatism. The pelvic region is abundantly supplied with blood from the point where the abdominal aorta divides, toning up the coccyx region and sacrum nerves. The entire body is kept in perfect equilibrium.

SAVASTIKA

The Auspicious Posture

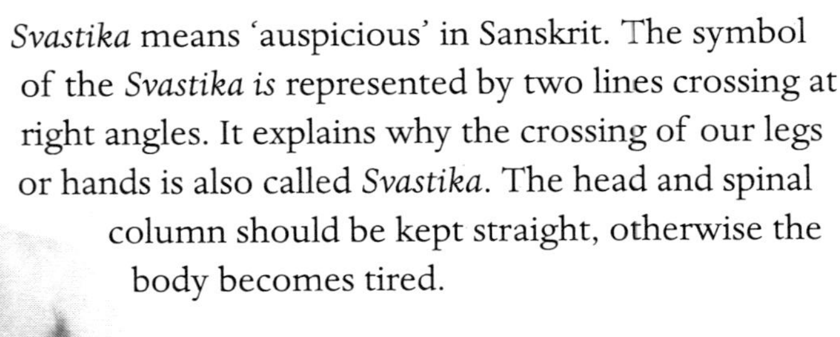

Svastika means 'auspicious' in Sanskrit. The symbol of the *Svastika is* represented by two lines crossing at right angles. It explains why the crossing of our legs or hands is also called *Svastika*. The head and spinal column should be kept straight, otherwise the body becomes tired.

TECHNIQUE

The right heel is placed against the left hip, and the left foot against the right calf. The hands are placed in one of the positions indicated in the description of the lotus position.

THERAPEUTIC ADVANTAGES

Identical to those of the lotus position.

SAMASANA

The Symmetrical Posture

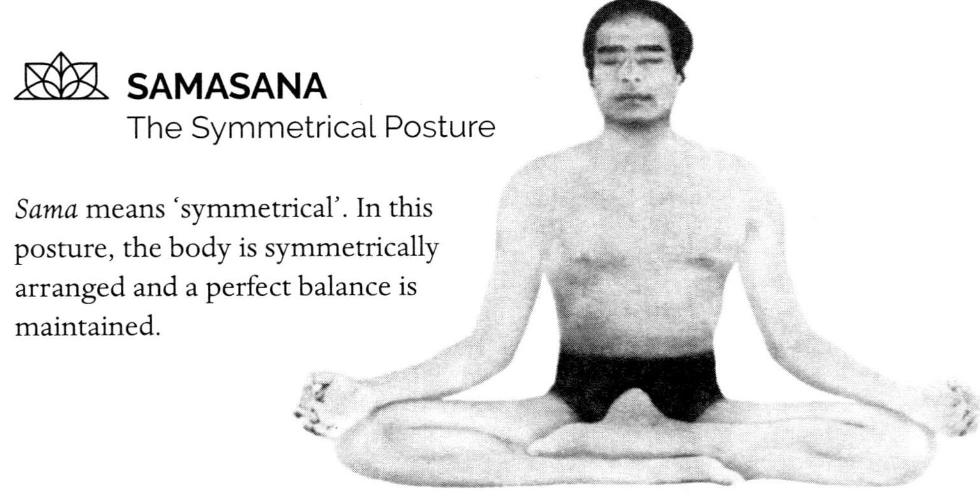

Sama means 'symmetrical'. In this posture, the body is symmetrically arranged and a perfect balance is maintained.

TECHNIQUE

Bend the left leg with the foot directly on the ground. Put the right foot on the left one placing the right heel against the pubic bone above the genital organs. This position may be reversed.

The position of the head, back and hands is the same as in the lotus position.

THERAPEUTIC ADVANTAGES

Same as in the lotus position.

SUKHASANA
Comfortable Posture

TECHNIQUE

Those who have difficulty in meditating in the Padmasana (lotus), Siddhasana (adept) or other meditation postures, may simply sit cross-legged. It is very important to keep the head and body straight, resting the hands on the knees without straining.

THERAPEUTIC ADVANTAGES

Identical to those gained in other meditation postures.

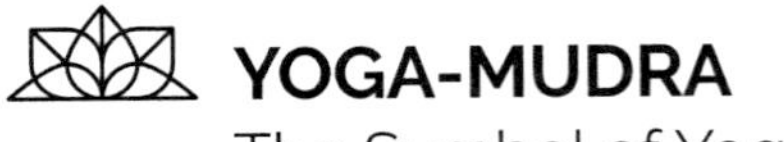

YOGA-MUDRA

The Symbol of Yoga

Mudra means 'symbol'.

The Mudras are special techniques which consist of the practice of Asanas, breath regulation, contraction exercises, and concentration to attain full control over the senses and perception.

A few of the more important Mudras, useful in maintaining perfect health, are given here. When practised for spiritual reasons, Yoga-Mudra helps to awaken the Kundalini.

TECHNIQUE

The exercise is practised in the Padmasana position. It may also be performed on or between the heels.

Place the hands behind the back, taking the left wrist in the right hand whilst keeping the spinal column perfectly upright. Inhale as in complete Yogic breathing and exhale slowly, gradually leaning forwards until the forehead touches the floor.

Stay in this position for as long as one feels comfortable, but without breathing. Direct the attention towards the abdominal region. Then while slowly breathing in, sit upright and relax. Repeat two or three times.

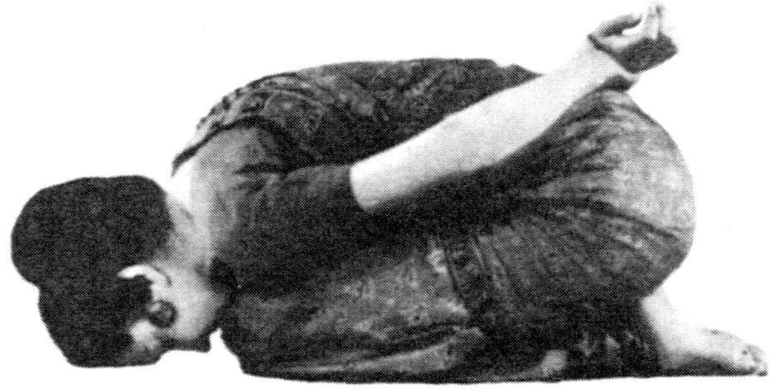

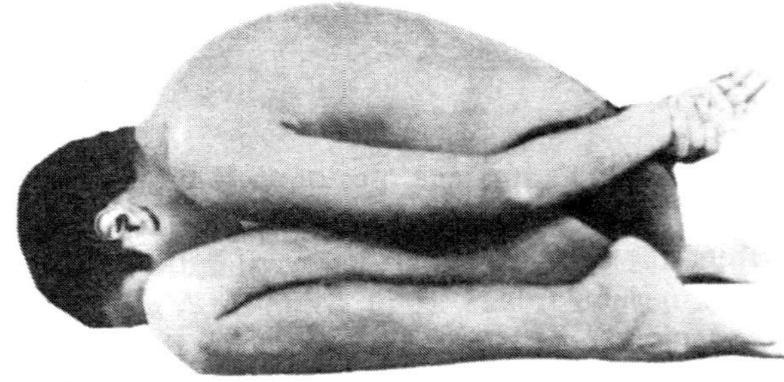

PRECAUTIONS

Lean forwards gently, without straining or jerking the spinal column.

THERAPEUTIC ADVANTAGES

This exercise is a remedy for constipation. It strengthens the abdominal muscles, and keeps the abdominal organs in their proper place. The entire nervous system, particularly the sacrolumbar nerves, are toned up. This Asana helps prevent sperm deficiency.

BADDHA KONASANA

Yoga-Mudra Feet Joined

PRECAUTIONS

Same as for Yoga-Mudra.

TECHNIQUE

Sit on the ground and join the soles of the feet. Spread the knees as far apart as possible. Inhale as in complete Yogic breathing whilst keeping the back straight. Exhale, and in so doing slip the forearms under the legs and hold the feet between the hands, elbows on the ground; then bend forwards slowly until the forehead touches the feet. Hold this position for several seconds before slowly sitting up again, inhaling deeply in the process. Relax by lying on the back.

Repeat this Asana two or three times. During the exercise, the 'consciousness' should be directed towards the abdominal region.

THERAPEUTIC EFFECT

This exercise is extremely beneficial to women. It regularizes menstrual disorders and ensures better functioning of the ovaries. The abdomen and back are stimulated by an abundant supply of blood, the kidneys and bladder are kept in good health. This posture is particularly recommended for those suffering from urinary complaints.

SUPTA-VAJRASANA

The Supine Pelvis Posture

PRECAUTIONS

Particular attention should be paid to the ankles and knees, and care should be taken not to force the joints.

TECHNIQUE

Sit on the ground between the heels. Hold the feet with the hands and lean slowly backwards, supporting oneself by the elbows, until the back and head are resting on the ground. Place the hands under the nape of the neck and practice complete Yogic breathing, keeping the body completely relaxed. Stay in this position for as long as it feels comfortable and direct the attention to the solar plexus. Then sit up again supporting oneself on the elbows, stretch out the legs and relax.

THERAPEUTIC ADVANTAGES

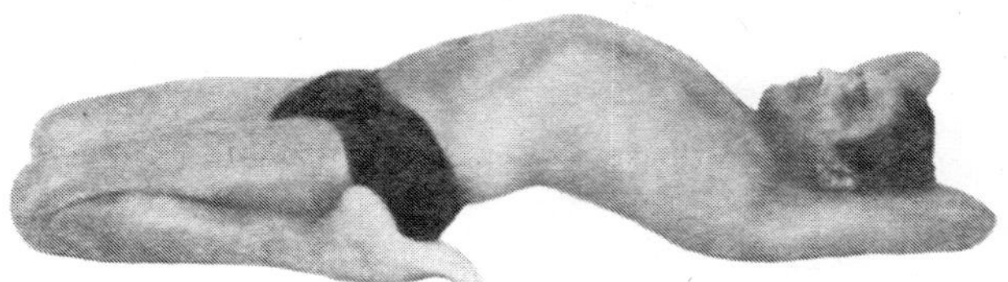

This is an excellent exercise for the ankles, knees and thighs. It is recommended for those who lack vital energy or whose glands are sluggish or who suffer from constipation, because this Asana makes the blood flow into the trunk of the body, stimulating and regenerating the solar plexus. It also tones up the subcutaneous nerves.

ARDHA-MATSYENDRASANA

Simplified Version of the Yogi Matsyendra Posture

This Asana is named after Yogi Matsyendra. Ardha means 'half'.

As Matsyendrasana is difficult to perform, it has been simplified and adopted as Ardha-Matsyendrasana.

PRECAUTIONS

Care must be taken not to force the elbows too much. During the exercise the back must remain straight. The spinal twist must be executed as smoothly as possible.

TECHNIQUE

Place the left heel under the right thigh and cross the right leg over the left thigh with the right foot flat on the ground. Catch hold of the big toe of the right foot with the left hand passing the arm in front of the right knee. Slowly turn the

head and back to the right stretching the right arm out behind and placing the right palm on the ground.

Breathe regularly directing the attention to the spinal column. Remain in the posture for a moment, then begin the other way round.

THERAPEUTIC ADVANTAGES

Swami Kuvalayananda writes in his book, *Asanas*, that we should exercise the spinal column in all possible directions if we wish to keep it in perfect health.

There are six ways of bending the spinal column: forwards, backwards, to both sides, and twisting to the left and right. Sarvangasana, Halasana, Paschimottanasana and Yoga-Mudra strengthen the spinal column by bending it forwards. Matsyasana, Bhujangasana, Salabhasana and Dhanurasana make it more flexible by bending it backwards.

Ardha-Matsyendrasana transmits to the spinal column two sideways twists; one to the left and other to the right. It is, therefore, a very useful Asana. It has great curative value and corrects spinal deformities; it has a beneficial effect on the gall-bladder, spleen, kidneys and bowels.

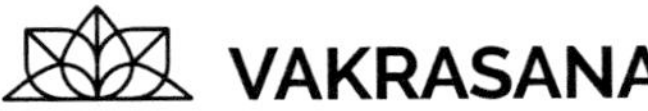

VAKRASANA

SPINAL TWIST

In Sanskrit, *Vakra* means 'twist'. Vakrasana was introduced into Hatha Yoga by

Swami Kuvalayananda. It is a simplified variation of Ardha-Matsyendrasana, designed for those who have stiff knees and find it difficult to bend them.

TECHNIQUE

Sitting on the ground with the legs stretched out, bend the right leg, bringing it up to the abdomen. Lift the right foot, pass it over the left thigh and rest it flat on the floor. Take the big toe of the right foot in the left hand, passing the arm in front of the right knee. Stretch out the right arm behind the back, with the palm of the hand flat on the ground. Remain in this position for several seconds, then repeat it the other way round. The attention should be directed towards the spinal column during the practice of this Asana.

THERAPEUTIC ADVANTAGES

Same as for Ardha-Matsyendrasana.

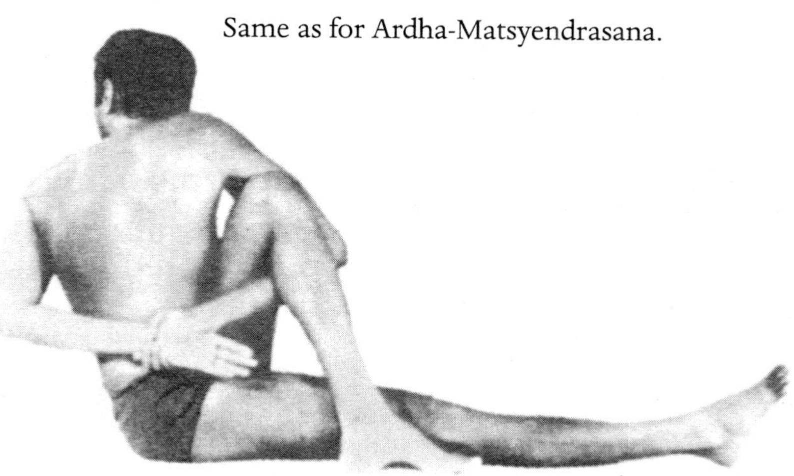

TRIKONASANA
Triangle Posture

TECHNIQUE

Stand with the legs apart. Inhale as in complete Yogic breathing whilst raising the arms bringing them up to a horizontal position.

Begin to exhale, bending the trunk to the right until the fingers of the right hand are touching the ground behind the right foot. The arms should form a vertical line, with the face turned upwards. After a few seconds, stand up again inhaling at the same time. Perform the same movement to the left, and finish the exercise by exhaling and slowly lowering the arms. Direct the attention to the spinal column. Repeat the Asana several times.

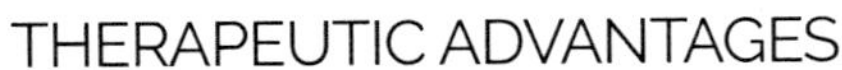

THERAPEUTIC ADVANTAGES

This Asana tones up the muscles in the back, the hips and legs, and prevents dislocation of the hip bones. It soothes the neck and back aches, and makes the legs more flexible.

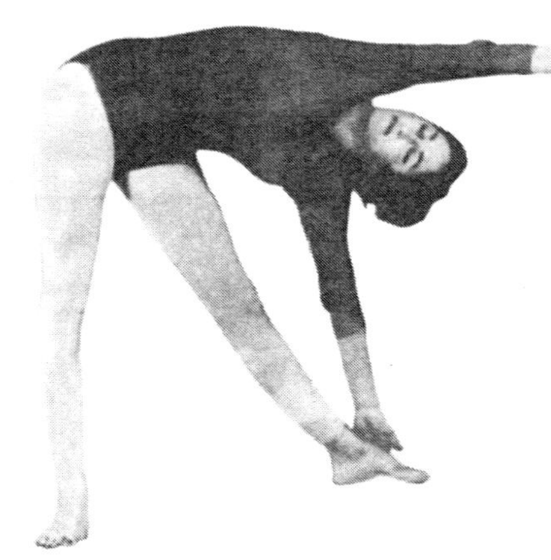

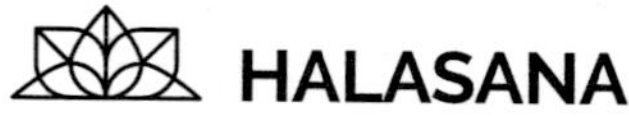

HALASANA
The Plough Posture

In Sanskrit, *Hala* means 'plough'.

TECHNIQUE

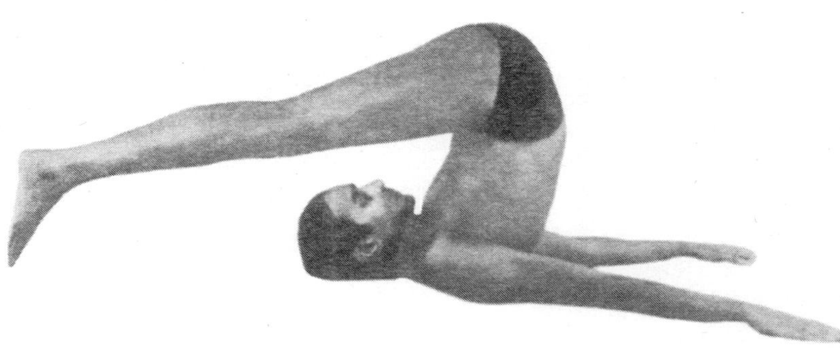

Lie on the back with the arms stretched by the side of the body, palms flat on the ground.

Inhale as in complete Yogic breathing. Exhale and slowly raise the legs stretched vertically. Supporting oneself by the arms flat on the ground, gently lower the legs behind the head until the tips of the feet are touching the ground. Remain in this position for several seconds breathing regularly. This marks the end of the first stage. For the second stage, push the feet a little further behind the head and stay in that position for several seconds breathing normally. To pass on to the third stage, push the feet even further back. In doing so, fold the arms and place the hands under the back of the neck. Hold this position for several seconds without forcing. Direct the attention to the spinal column while executing the three stages.

To return to the starting position, place the arms along the body, gradually bring the feet up towards the head, passing through the first two stages the other way round and raise the legs to a vertical position before dropping them gently onto the ground and relaxing.

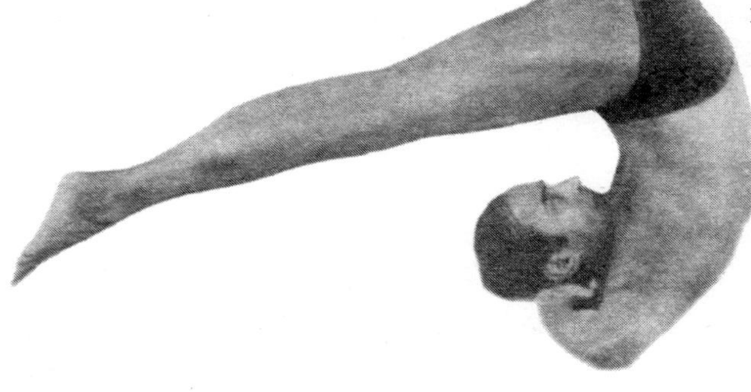

Each stage exercises the spinal column differently.

PRECAUTIONS

Those who have a stiff spinal column should practise this Asana with great care, without ever straining, and avoiding all brusque movements. If practised regularly and persistently, this exercise will make even the stiffest spine flexible. Viparitakarani is a good preparation for Halasana.

THERAPEUTIC ADVANTAGES

This Asana is extremely beneficial to the spinal column. The whole region receives an abundant supply of blood which revitalizes the nerves and muscles of the back. Exhaustion or any fatigue quickly disappear. The position also has a regenerating effect on the glandular system, and clears up menstrual disorders. When practised regularly, the exercise prevents fat from forming on the stomach, hips and waist.

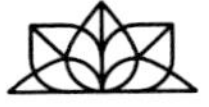

PASCHIMOTTANASANA

Stretching the Back and Hips

TECHNIQUE

Stretch out on the back with feet together. Raise the arms above the head inhaling as in complete Yogic breathing. Sit up and exhale while leaning forwards until the head touches the knees, which should remain flat. Hold the big toe of the right foot with the thumb and index finger of the right hand, and the big toe of the left foot with the thumb and index finger of the left hand. An

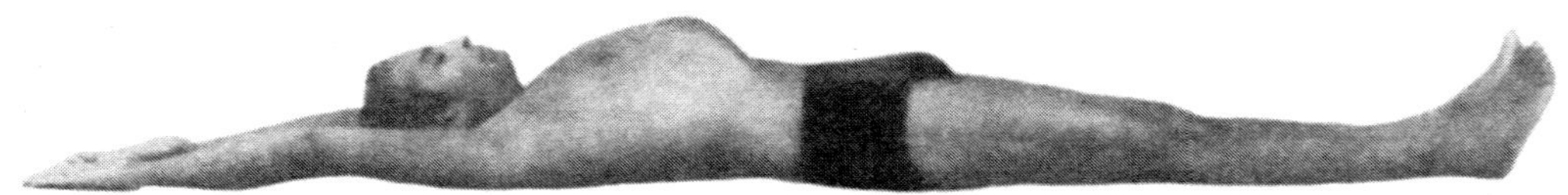

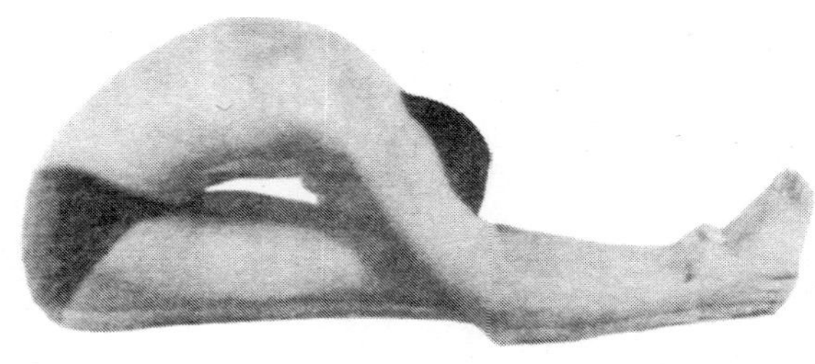

alternative is simply to hold the ankles in each hand, with the elbows on the floor. Stay in this position for several seconds, then inhale deeply whilst gradually sitting up. Stretch out on the back, hands resting beside the body. Exhale and relax. While the Asana is being performed direct the attention to the abdominal region.

PRECAUTIONS

In leaning forward, the knees must remain flat to allow the muscles or the legs and sacrolumbar region to be fully stretched. All brusque movements are to be avoided and one should not strain or force. Even if at the beginning one finds it difficult to lean forward, a little patience and perseverance will help get rid of all stiffness.

THERAPEUTIC ADVANTAGES

When practiced in moderation (three minutes a day maximum, otherwise the effect is reversed), Paschimottanasana is a good remedy for constipation. All the posterior back muscles are stretched to their fullest extent and the abdominal muscles are strengthened, thus preventing the formation of fat around the stomach. This Asana has a particularly salutary effect on the spinal column. Blood rushes to the gonads, prostate gland, uterus and bladder, to improve their state of health.
The posture regenerates the kidneys and digestive organs. It can check and prevent diabetes.

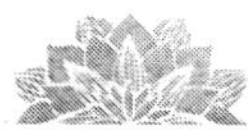

OURDHVA PASCHIMOTTANASANA

Stretching the Back and Legs Upwards

Ourdhva means 'upwards'.

TECHNIQUE

Lie on the back. Bend the knees and hold the feet in the hands. Inhale as in complete Yogic breathing, then exhale and unbend the legs vertically until they are completely straight. Bring the head near the knees and maintain the .position for several seconds. Then bend the knees, lower the legs and relax.

PRECAUTIONS

Same as for Paschimottanasana.

THERAPEUTIC ADVANTAGES

Similar to those of Paschimottanasana, but this is also an exercise for equilibrium and mental stability which develops the powers of concentration.

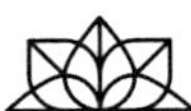

PADAHASTASANA

Stretching the Back and Legs Downwards

In Sanskrit *Pada* means 'foot' and *Hasta* 'hand'.

TECHNIQUE

Stand with the feet together, and arms beside the body. Inhale as in complete Yogic breathing, then exhale. In so doing, lean slowly

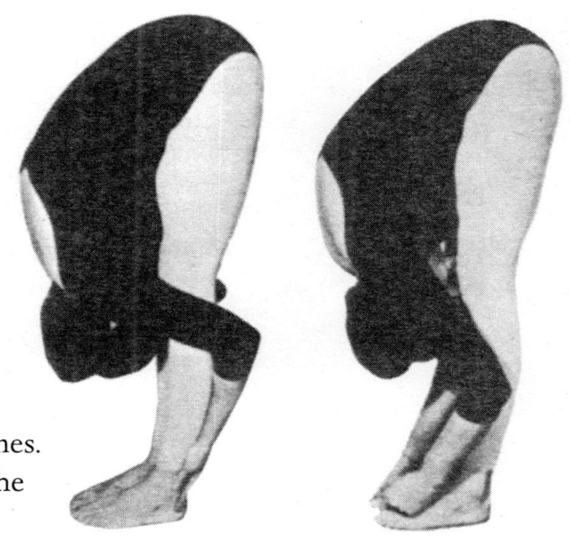

forwards — without stooping — and hold the foot with the hand, or the big toe with the index finger and thumb (as for Paschimottanasana). Now touch the knees with the head, keeping the legs straight. Stay like this for several seconds, then slowly stand up breathing in deeply, and relax. Repeat the exercise two or three times. While executing the Asana, direct the attention to the abdominal region.

PRECAUTIONS

Sudden movements of the spinal column are to be avoided.

THERAPEUTIC ADVANTAGES

This exercise tones up the organs in the abdomen, and ensures the proper functioning of the liver and spleen. It is excellent for those suffering from digestive troubles.

Like Paschimottanasana, this Asana has a beneficial effect on the spinal column, allowing the muscles in the back and legs to be stretched to their fullest extent.

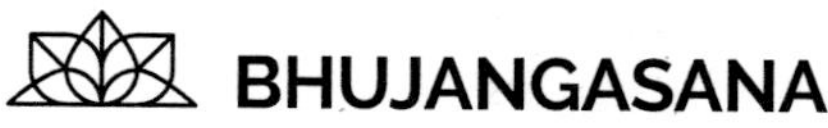

BHUJANGASANA
The Cobra Position

TECHNIQUE

Lie on the stomach, with palms on the ground underneath the shoulders. Inhale as in complete Yogic breathing. Supporting

oneself lightly on the arms, slowly raise the head and trunk, leaning backwards as far as possible, but without raising the abdominal region from the ground. Hold this position for several seconds; then exhale slowly and gradually return to the starting position. Relax by putting the hands underneath the forehead. Repeat the exercise two or three times.

PRECAUTIONS

Those who have a stiff spinal column should start slowly and carefully. Sudden movements are to be avoided.

THERAPEUTIC ADVANTAGES

During the practice of Bhujangasana, the muscles of the back come into play, exerting pressure on the vertebrae from the neck down to the lower part of the spinal column, and provoking a copious supply of blood to this region, thus toning it up.

This Asana may correct discs that have slipped slightly. It soothes backaches, renders the spinal column more flexible and keeps it in good health.

The exercise also has a beneficial effect on the kidneys (adrenal glands), and simulates digestion.

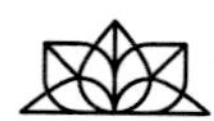

ARDHA-BHUJANGASANA

Simplified Cobra Position

TECHNIQUE

Touch the ground with the left knee and put the right foot out in front so that the tibia (the larger bone in the lower leg) remains vertical. Inhale as in complete Yogic breathing. While exhaling, move the weight of the body forwards, without bending the torso, until the fingers are touching the ground. The arms should remain vertical throughout the exercise. Remain in this pose for several seconds without breathing, then slowly rise while inhaling in the complete Yogic breathing manner. Repeat two or three times and carry out the same exercise with the other leg. Then relax. While the Asana is being performed, concentrate on the movement.

THERAPEUTIC ADVANTAGES

This Asana maintains the body's equilibrium. It has a beneficial effect on the kidneys and prevents the formation of fat around the hips. The exercise makes the spinal column, the legs and ankles more flexible.

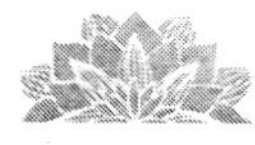

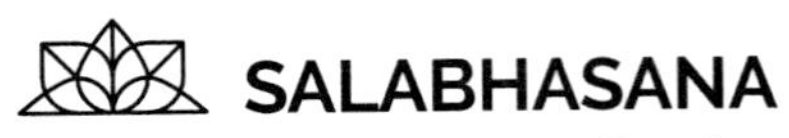

SALABHASANA

The Locust Posture

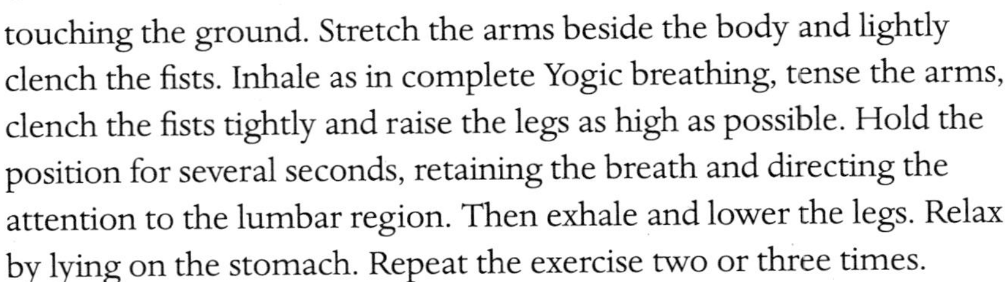

TECHNIQUE

Lie on stomach, with chin or forehead touching the ground. Stretch the arms beside the body and lightly clench the fists. Inhale as in complete Yogic breathing, tense the arms, clench the fists tightly and raise the legs as high as possible. Hold the position for several seconds, retaining the breath and directing the attention to the lumbar region. Then exhale and lower the legs. Relax by lying on the stomach. Repeat the exercise two or three times.

PRECAUTIONS

Do not tire lungs by prolonging posture or raising legs brusquely.

THERAPEUTIC ADVANTAGES

An excellent exercise for muscles in back, arms and abdomen. It fortifies the latter and has a beneficial effect on the digestive organs, curing stubborn constipation. This Asana brings a large supply of blood to the kidneys, thus cleaning and, regenerating them.

ARDHA-SALABHASANA

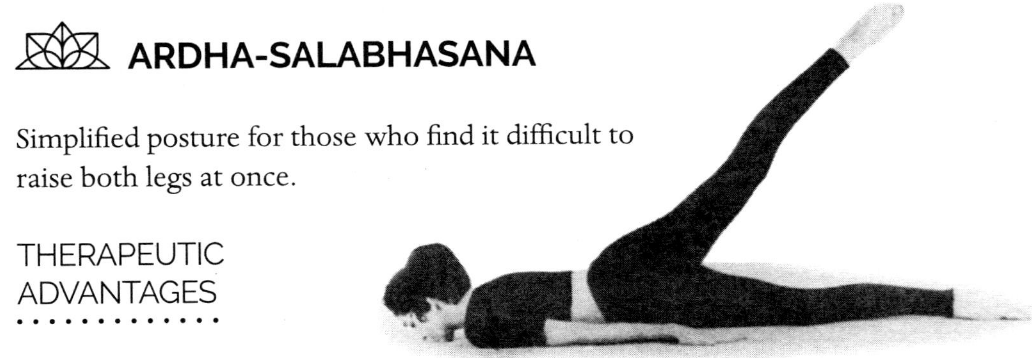

Simplified posture for those who find it difficult to raise both legs at once.

THERAPEUTIC ADVANTAGES

Same as for Salabhasana.

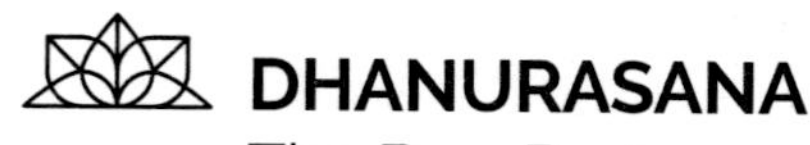

DHANURASANA

The Bow Posture

In Sanskrit, *Dhanus* means 'bow'.

TECHNIQUE

Lie on the stomach. Bend the knees whilst keeping them together. Take the ankles in the hands and rest the chin on the ground. Inhale as in complete Yogic breathing, then raise the legs, head and upper part of the body whilst arching the back. Remain in this position as long as possible, breathing regularly and directing the attention to the lower part of the spinal column (pelvic region). Now relax the body gradually and return to the original position. Repeat the exercise two or three times, then relax.

PRECAUTIONS

This exercise requires a certain amount of effort. Be careful of the joints, and above all, take it very easy.

THERAPEUTIC ADVANTAGES

This Asana loosens up the spinal column and strengthens the nervous centres. It also recharges the solar plexus with vital energy and tones up the abdominal organs. The exercise stimulates the endocrine glands and is excellent for women suffering from irregular or faulty menstruation. It also prevents fat from forming around the stomach and hips.

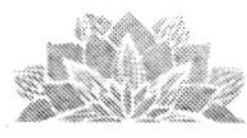

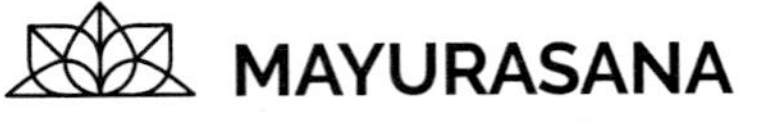

MAYURASANA

The Peacock Posture

TECHNIQUE

Kneel on the ground, knees apart, palms flat on the floor, fingers pointing towards the feet. Bring the elbows under the abdomen just under the navel, and lean forward to touch the ground with the forehead. Lean on it and stretch out the legs behind. Raise the feet and head, and keep the body in a position parallel to the ground (like a horizontal bar) supporting it entirely on the arms. Stay balanced in this posture for as long as possible, then lie on the stomach and relax. During this Asana, concentrate on the movement itself and breathe normally.

PRECAUTIONS

This is a very difficult Asana and should therefore be practised with great care. It requires very flexible hands and wrists, so watch out for the joints.

THERAPEUTIC ADVANTAGES

This posture requires great determination and concentration. It is an excellent way of bringing the body into equilibrium and fortifying the hands, wrists and forearms. Practice of this Asana will exert pressure inside the abdomen, thus toning up the organs and muscles in this area. The increased supply of blood to the digestive organs makes them healthier and cures constipation.

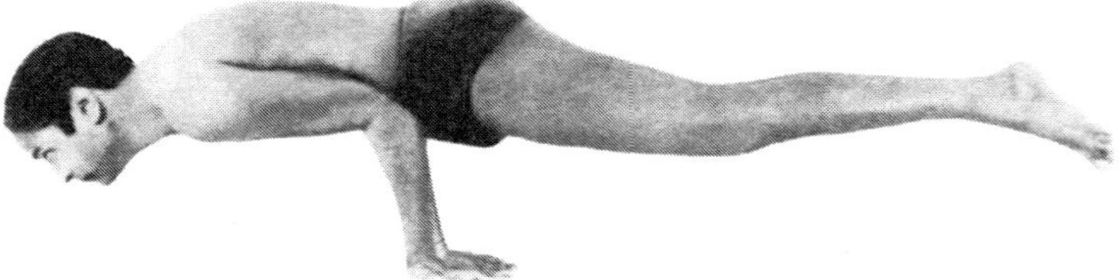

JALANDHARA BANDHA

Chin-Lock

Jala means 'net' and refers to the brain and nerves crossing the neck. *Dhara* signifies 'the action of pulling upwards' and Bandha 'contraction'.

During Jalandhara, the neck and throat are contracted and the chin locked into position above the hollow of the sternum (breast bone). This movement may be acquired by practising Sarvangasana.

TECHNIQNE

Sit in the Padmasana or Siddhasana position. Lower the head and bury the chin firmly in the hollow above the breast bone. This may be done at any time during breathing.

THERAPEUTIC ADVANTAGES

This exercise regulates the bloodstream and Prana flowing towards the heart, neck, glands, head and brain.

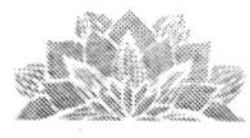

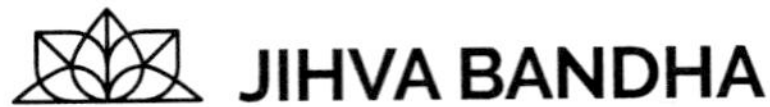

JIHVA BANDHA

Contraction of the Tongue or the Tongue-Lock

In Sanskrit, *Jihva* means 'tongue' and *Bandh* 'contraction'.

TECHNIQUE

This exercise should be practised in the lotus position or sitting cross-legged. Place the tongue on the interior of the upper jaw and press hard against the roof of the mouth. Open the mouth as wide as possible keeping the tongue in position (like a leech) for several seconds.

Variation: Put the tongue out as far as it will go, then gradually retract it into the throat, rolling the tip at the back, as if one were about to swallow it. Perform complete Yogic breathing three or four times after the exercise.

THERAPEUTIC ADVANTAGES

This Bandha exercises the neck muscles, improves the circulation of blood in this region of the body, as well as the hearing. It also has a beneficial effect on the nerves in the neck, the pharynx and larynx, the tonsils, thyroid and salivary glands.

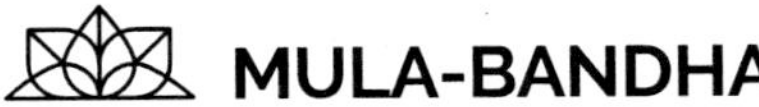

MULA-BANDHA

Contraction of the Pelvic and Anal Muscles

The Sanskrit word *Mula* means 'root' or 'source', and *Bandha* 'contraction'. In this posture the organs of the pelvic region are contracted and controlled.

TECHNIQUE

The posture may be carried out in Siddhasana or other Asanas, especially Paschimottanasana, Sarvangasana, Sirshasana or simply standing up straight. Inhale slowly, as in complete Yogic breathing. Hold the breath and contract the ring of muscles around the anus, thus causing the whole of the pelvic region to contract, i.e., the lower abdomen between the navel and the anus. Relax after a few moments, exhaling slowly. Repeat the exercise several times. During the execution of Mula-Bandha, direct the attention to the pelvic region. Mula-Bandha may also be performed with the lungs empty, i.e., after exhaling.

PRECAUTIONS

When carried out incorrectly, this Bandha can lead to chronic constipation, and may throw the digestive system out of order. As the genital organs are also involved, mistakes in execution can also cause serious disorders in this region. One should therefore proceed systematically and patiently. It is very dangerous to attempt this Bandha without the personal guidance of a trained guru.

THERAPEUTIC ADVANTAGES

The central nervous system and the sympathetic nerves are stimulated by the nerve-endings connected to the ring of muscles around the anus. Mula-Bandha also has a beneficial effect on the nerves situated in the lower part of the trunk. The pancreas and sexual glands are also regenerated.

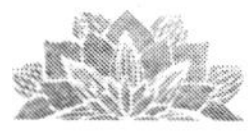

UDDIYANA-BANDHA

Raising of the Diaphragm

In Sanskrit *Uddiyana* means 'to raise' and *Bandha* 'contraction'.

TECHNIQUE

Stand with legs roughly 1 to 1½ feet apart, knees very slightly bent. Press hard on the thighs with the hands allowing the body to lean forward slightly and inhale as in complete Yogic breathing, then exhale slowly and deeply. Then bring the abdominal wall as far back towards the spinal column as possible, while raising the diaphragm as high as it will go. Hold this posture for a moment, then inhale slowly.

To begin with, repeat the exercise three to five times, gradually increasing the number until it is possible to perform the Asana at least twelve times.

PRECAUTIONS

Those suffering from serious abdominal complaints should not perform this exercise.

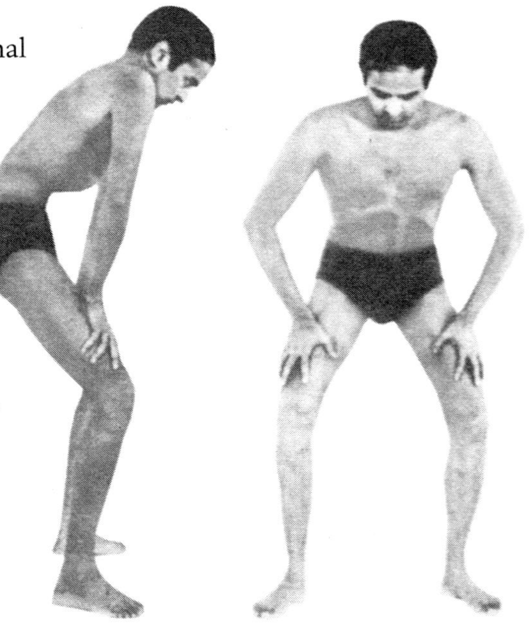

THERAPEUTIC ADVANTAGES

A sluggish colon may be set moving properly, constipation dyspepsia and liver trouble prevented. This exercise is also an excellent remedy against prolapses of the stomach uterus or intestines. It cures most gastric complaints and removes toxins from the digestive tract. The figure and waist will remain in shape, for this exercise prevents fat deposits from forming around the abdomen and waist.

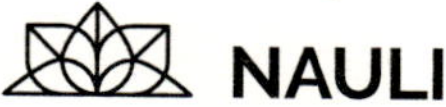

NAULI

Isolation of the Rectal Abdominal Muscles

TECHNIQUE

Stand with legs apart. Press on the thighs with the hands, as in Uddiyana-Bandha. After inhaling once as in complete Yogic breathing, exhale forcefully, and bring the abdominal wall back towards the interior. Now contract the central abdominal muscles and arch them by pushing strongly forwards. This is called Madhyama-Nauli (central isolation).

To perform uni-lateral isolation of the right and left muscles, lean slowly forward to the right and press hard on the right thigh with the

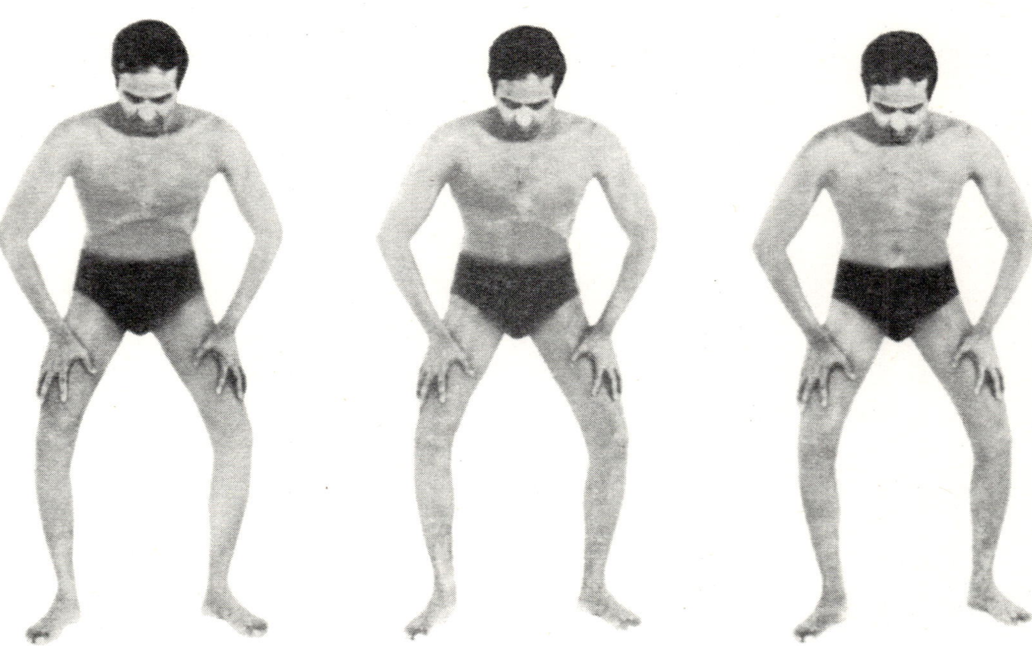

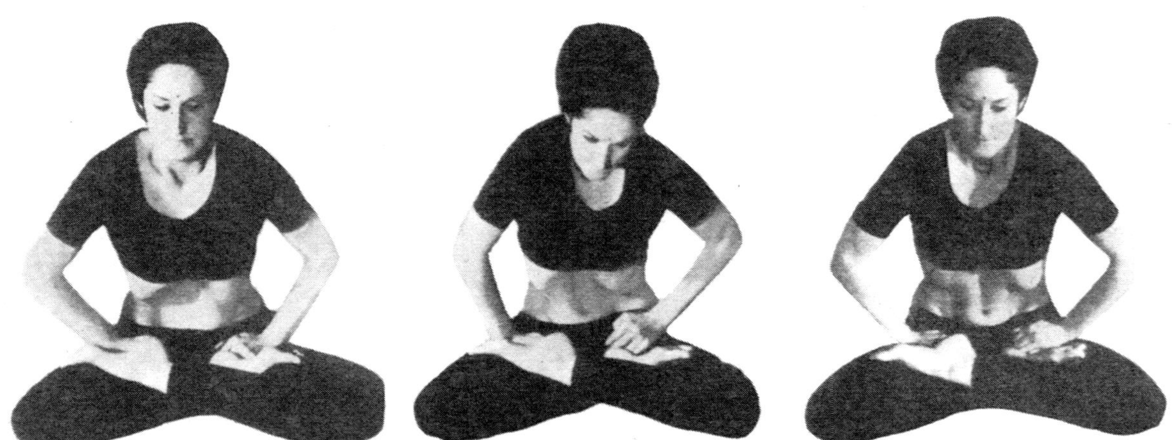

right hand, leaving the left hand loose. This is called Dakshina-Nauli (unilateral isolation right). When performed the other way round, i.e., on the left, it is called Varna-Nauli (unilateral isolation left).

The last variation of Nauli is the rotation of the muscles. The movements described above are transmitted in a circular rhythm to the rectal abdominal muscles in isolation. This circular movement may be obtained by slowly rotating the pelvis.

PRECAUTIONS

Same as for Uddiyana-Bandha. It should be perfomed under the guidance of a trained guru.

THERAPEUTIC ADVANTAGES

The abdominal muscles are strengthened and regenerated. All the organs in the abdomen are automatically massaged, thus stimulating their action.

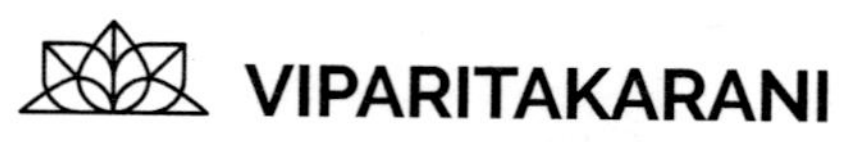

VIPARITAKARANI

The Inverted Posture

In Sanskrit, *Viparita* means 'inverted' and *Karani* 'action'.

This exercise is called Viparitakarani because when practised, the body takes up an inverted position, i.e., the legs above the head.

TECHNIQUE

Lie on the back and inhale as in complete Yogic breathing. Exhale and raise the legs and hips with the help of the arms. Bend the arms and hold the hips in the hands so that the body is supported on the elbows, shoulder-blades and head. The legs should form an angle of 60 to 70 degrees with the ground. Practise abdominal respiration and direct the attention to the thyroid gland. This position may be kept for as long as one feels comfortable. To finish, lower the legs gently to the ground and relax in the starting position. Repeat the exercise two or three times.

PRECAUTIONS

Those with high blood pressure should consult an experienced Yoga instructor. Before performing this Asana, one should completely relax.

THERAPEUTIC ADVANTAGES

Hatha-Yoga considers the inverted position to be the most important exercise for reviving the body. The three main inverted postures are Viparitakarani, Sarvangasana and Sirshasana. Viparitakarani is the easiest of the three to execute and has the

advantage of combining the therapeutic effects of the other two, but in a milder form. It is nevertheless highly recommended for recharging the body with new energy.

In this position, the blood flows abundantly to the neck, throat and head, so that the thyroid and pituitary glands plus the nervous centres of the brain, are all regenerated. The pose also prevents formation of wrinkles and can cure goitres.

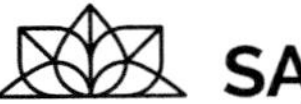

SARVANGASANA
Shoulder-Stand

In Sanskrit, *Sarva* means 'entire' or 'whole' and *Anga* 'body'.

TECHNIQUE

Lie on the back and relax completely. Inhale as in complete Yogic breathing, then whilst exhaling slowly, raise the legs, hips and trunk in a continuous movement until vertical. Raise the legs (knees straight) and hips by supporting the arms on the ground; then bend the elbows and hold the trunk in the hands. In this posture the chin is buried in the sternum (upper chest). Practise abdominal respiration and retain the position for as long as is comfortable. Direct the attention to the thyroid gland.

To return to the starting position, gently lower the trunk, pelvis and legs, and relax on the ground. Repeat the exercise two or three times.

PRECAUTIONS

All the precautions indicated for Viparitakarani apply to this Asana as well.

THERAPEUTIC ADVANTAGES

It is a known fact that our state of health depends, to a large extent, on the proper functioning of the thyroid gland. In this posture, the thyroid receives an abundant supply of fresh blood. Owing to the regenerating effect of Sarvangasana on the thyroid, one is kept in perfect health. Regular practice of the Asana will make the symptoms of premature aging, produced by thyroid disorders, completely disappear. One regains youthful vigour, wrinkles soften, and the body stays supple to a very great age.

This posture is also a blessing to those with ovary problems and ensures the good functioning of the sexual glands, both male and female. The shoulder-stand clears congestion in the legs, and has a salutary effect on veins and haemorroids.

Owing to its regenerative effect on the nervous system, Sarvangasana and indeed Sirshasana can cure insomnia and depression. The only difference between Sarvangasana and Sirshasana is in the position of the head. Hence the first has more effect on the thyroid, while the second influences the brain. As both of these Asanas require the body to be in a vertical position, the therapeutic effects of Sarvangasana are also produced by Sirshasana, since the position is similar.

ARDHA-SARVANGASANA

Modified Shoulder-stand

This posture is particularly suited to those with a weak back. By bending the knees, the muscles in the back are partly relaxed.

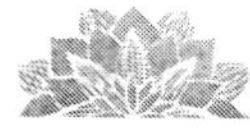

TECHNIQUE

Adopt the Sarvangasana pose, but once the trunk and legs are positioned vertically, bend and lower the knees until the thighs are parallel to the ground.

THERAPEUTIC ADVANTAGES

Similar to those of Sarvangasana.

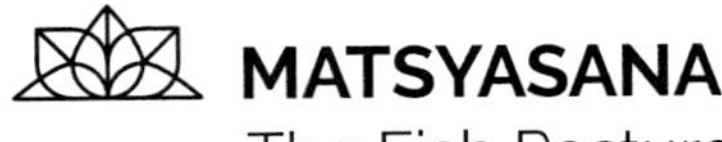

MATSYASANA
The Fish Posture

The Sanskrit word *Matsya* signifies 'fish'.

This posture is called Matsyasana because it allows those who execute it carefully to float on the surface of water, like a fish, for quite some time.

It is recommended to practise this Asana after Sarvangasana (shoulder-stand) to obtain excellent therapeutic results.

TECHNIQUE

Sit in the Padmasana (lotus) position and inhale as in complete Yogic breathing. Exhale and, with the help of the elbows, lean the trunk backwards. Lift the chest upwards and rest the crown of the head on the ground. Take hold of the big toes. Breathe lightly and direct the attention to the thyroid gland. Hold the posture for several seconds, then return to the starting position. Relax lying on the back.

PRECAUTIONS

If the lotus position is too difficult, this Asana may be performed sitting cross-legged.

THERAPEUTIC ADVANTAGES

This exercise enlarges the thoracic cage and allows deeper breathing. It renders the neck supple and removes all aches and stiffness. The neck muscles are fully stretched, thus provoking an abundant flow of blood to this region of the body, and regenerating the thyroid and tonsils. This Asana also fortifies the muscles in the back and has a beneficial effect on the spinal column.

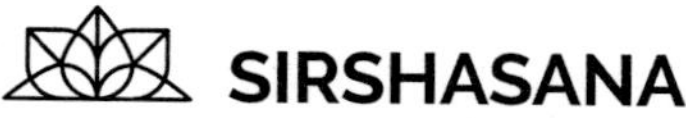

SIRSHASANA
Head-Stand

In Sanskrit, *Sirsh* means 'head'.

TECHNIQUE

Adopt a kneeling position and rest the forearms on the ground in front. Join the hands and interlace the fingers; place them on the head so that the section between the crown and the forehead is touching the ground. Raise the hips and gently bring the feet nearer the head, so that the torso may be lifted. Raise the feet by bending the knees then stretch the legs until the whole body forms a vertical line. Breathe regularly and direct the attention to the brain. Remain in this posture for as long as one feels comfortable. To come down, bend the knees, then the body at the hips, lower the legs until the feet and knees are touching the ground. Relax in the starting

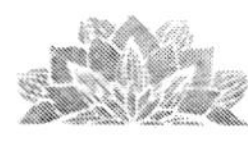

position, but support the head by placing the fists one on top of the other between the forehead and the ground.

At the beginning, this posture should be held for a maximum of 5 seconds, then the time may be increased by 5 seconds a week, up to 3 minutes.

PRECAUTIONS

Those with high blood pressure, a weak heart, fragile eye capillaries or earache should not practise this Asana.

If, for any particular reason, one is unable to perform this posture, there is no need for worry — Viparitakarani and Sarvangasana may be performed in its place since their therapeutic effects are similar.

Sirshasana should never be carried out after strenous exercise.

THERAPEUTIC ADVANTAGES

All our activities, whether physical or mental, are governed by the brain. The nervous system spreads throughout the organism and is either directly or indirectly connected to it. Hence the abundant influx of arterial blood to the brain caused by Sirshasana regenerates both the brain and the complete nervous system. For the same reason, this Asana ensures good health to the sensorial

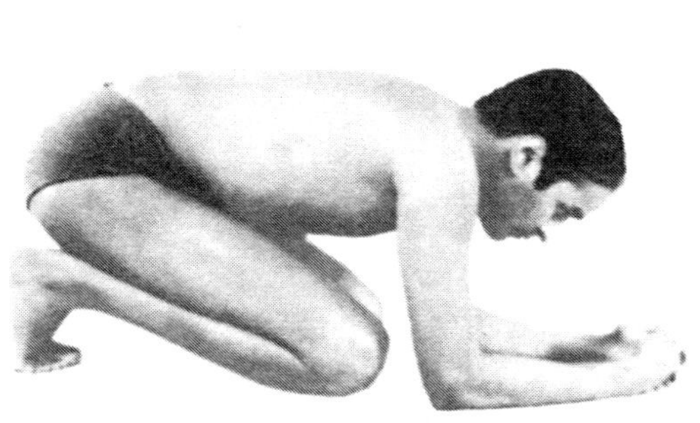

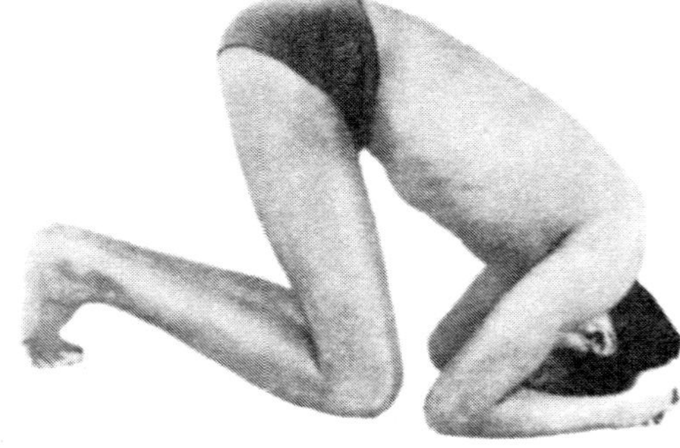

organs, whose functioning depends on the various brain centres. It develops the mental faculties, e.g., the memory and powers of concentration, and even encourages some of the 'occult' faculties, such as clairvoyance and telepathy.

This exercise also has a beneficial effect on the endocrine and digestive systems. It cures a congested liver and spleen, allowing the blood to circulate freely in these organs. Nervous asthma may also be soothed by this Asana.

Practice of Sirshasana provides us with a feeling of equilibrium and well-being. It ensures perfect health, which is why Yogis call it 'the king of Asanas'.

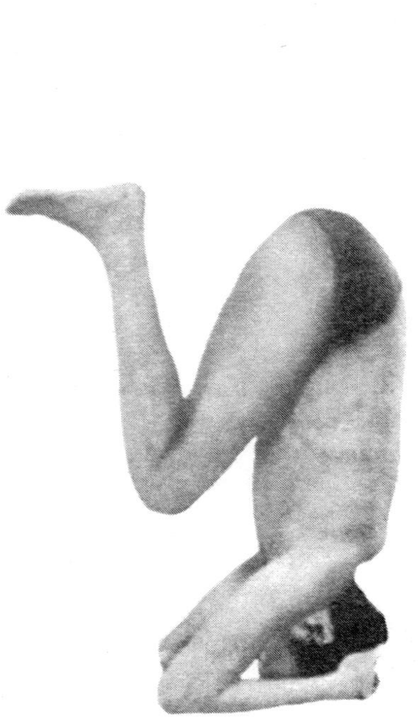

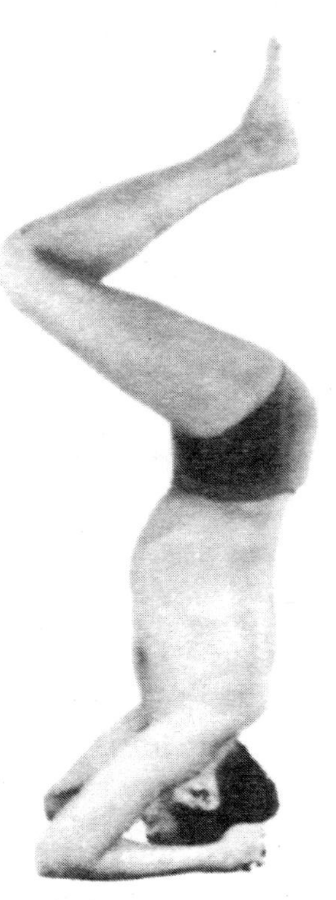

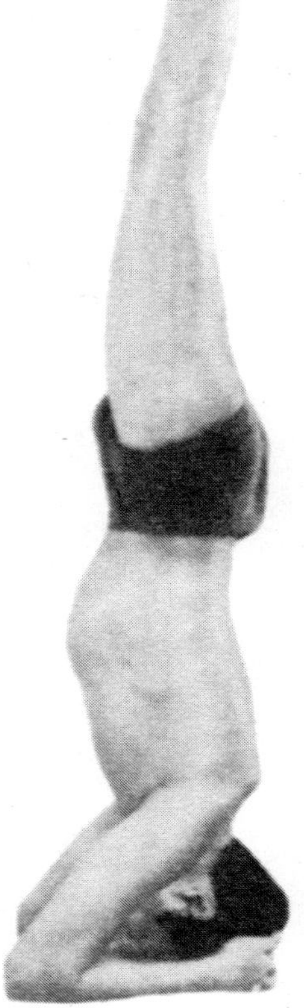

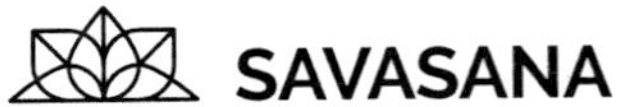

SAVASANA

Complete Relaxation Posture

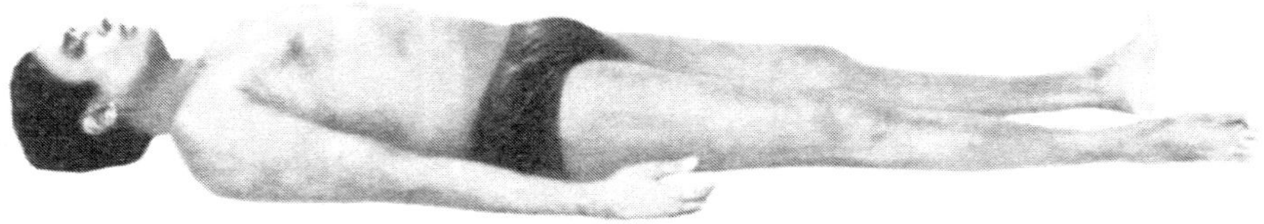

In Sanskrit, *Sava* means 'corpse'.

This posture derives its name from the fact that one lies on the back like a corpse, with mind and body totally relaxed.

TECHNIQUE

Lie on the back, with arms at the sides, legs stretched out and slightly apart. Close the eyes and breathe slowly and deeply, as in complete Yogic breathing. Begin by consciously and gradually relaxing each part and each muscle of the body: feet, calves, knees, thighs, abdomen, hips, back, hands, arms, shoulders, neck, head and face. One should let oneself go completely, like a cat when it relaxes, letting the muscles go. It should seem as though one can no longer feel the body.

Next, one should try and forget all external thoughts, so that the brain becomes empty.

Breathing should be completely rhythmical — inhaling and exhaling taking the same time — the regularity of the breath is absolutely essential to complete relaxation. Once one has settled down into an individual rhythm, one should concentrate on absorbing a flow of calm at each breath. To achieve such mental relaxation, the attention should be directed to the breathing. By consciously immobilizing the mind and body, and breathing properly, one learns how to find true relaxation; one feels filled with rest, peace and plenitude.

THERAPEUTIC ADVANTAGES

Often a tensed body and irregular breathing are the cause of bad health. Rhythmic breathing in Savasana is, therefore, extremely salutary for the entire body, provided it is taught properly by an instructor. By resting in this way, one avoids all mental stress. The heart and nervous system are calmed, and the circulation becomes regular.

After a few minutes' relaxation in Savasana, the whole organism is recharged with Prana, i.e., renewed energy and regenerative force. A quarter of an hour's rest of this kind eliminates the toxins that have accumulated in the blood.

Experiments performed at the Yoga Research Institute, Lonavla, have proved that it is possible, by Yogic relaxation, to cure high blood pressure, insomnia, nervous disorders and certain types of nervous depression.

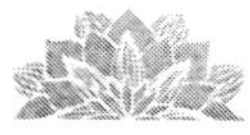

4

Asanas for Equilibrium, Concentration and Mental Stability

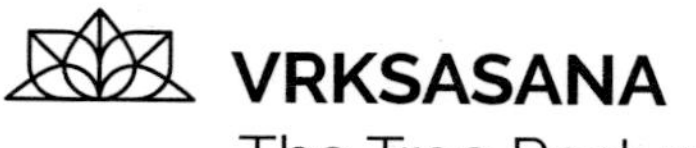

VRKSASANA
The Tree Posture

This Asana not only helps establish equilibrium and mental stability, but also makes the knee joints more supple.

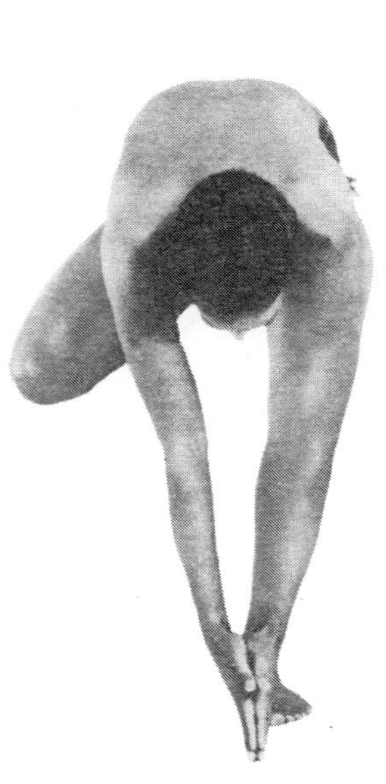

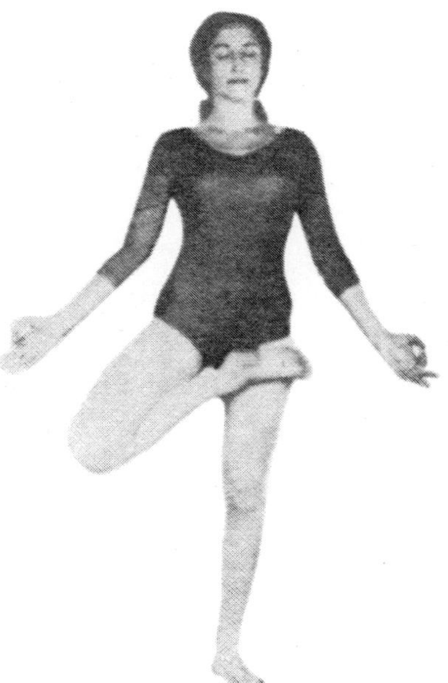

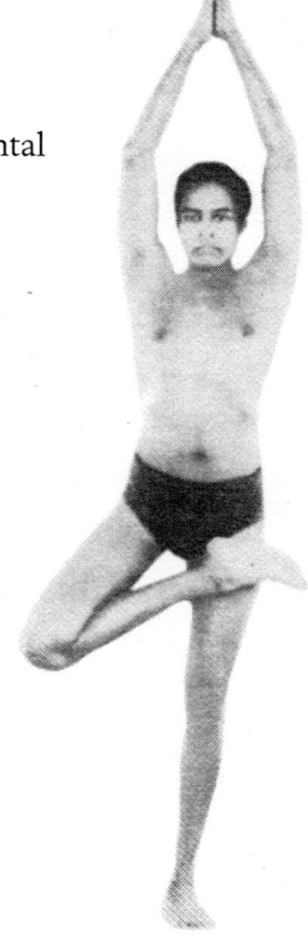

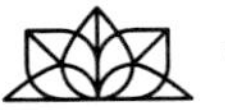

VATYANASANA

The Horse's Head Posture

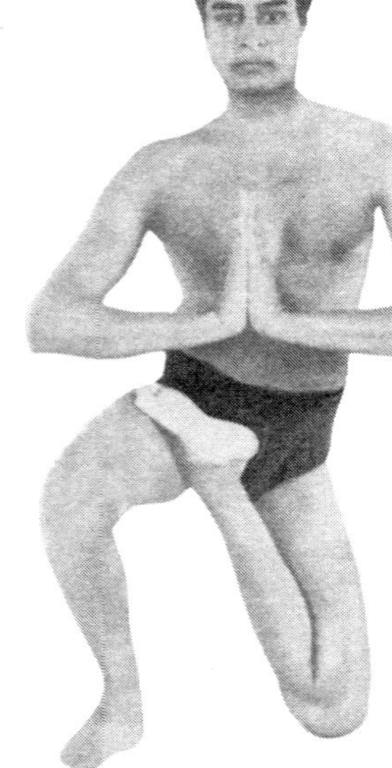

The posture renders the knees and feet more supple, fortifies the legs and prevents certain kinds of rheumatism.

UTTHITA HASTA PADANGUSTHASANA

Foot-Holding Posture

Phase 1: Stand with legs slightly apart.

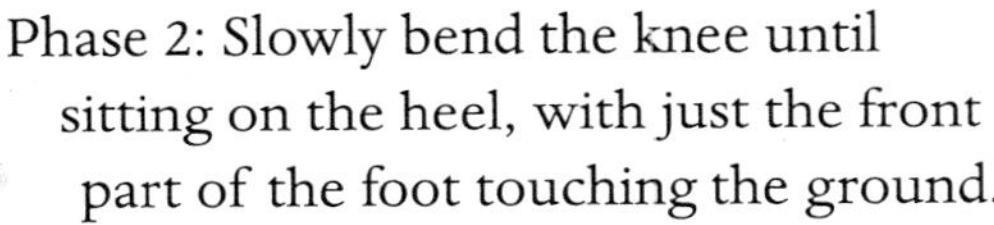

Phase 2: Slowly bend the knee until sitting on the heel, with just the front part of the foot touching the ground.

This posture fortifies the leg muscles.

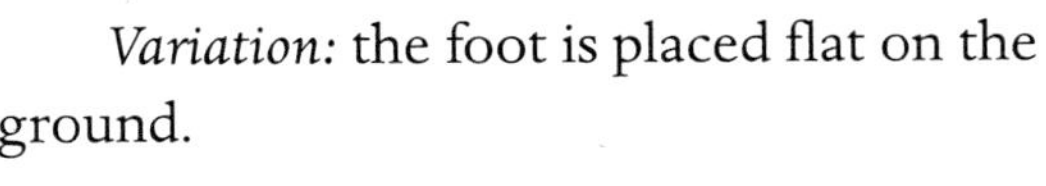

Variation: the foot is placed flat on the ground.

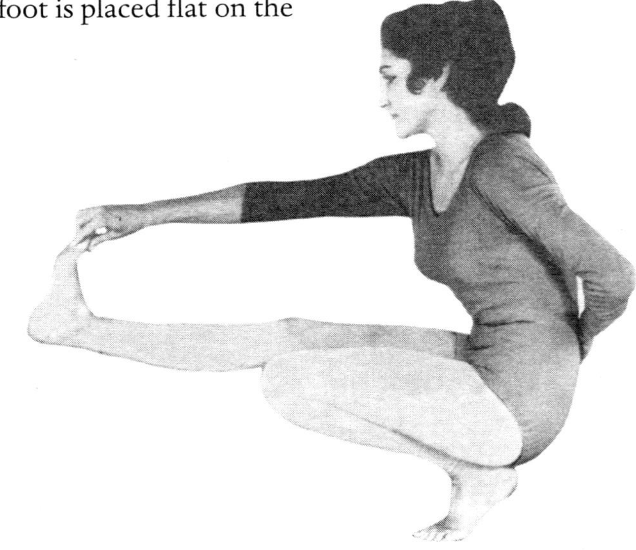

BAKASANA

The Crow Posture

This Asana reinforces the arm and shoulder muscles, strengthens the wrists and irrigates the blood vessels in the neck and face.

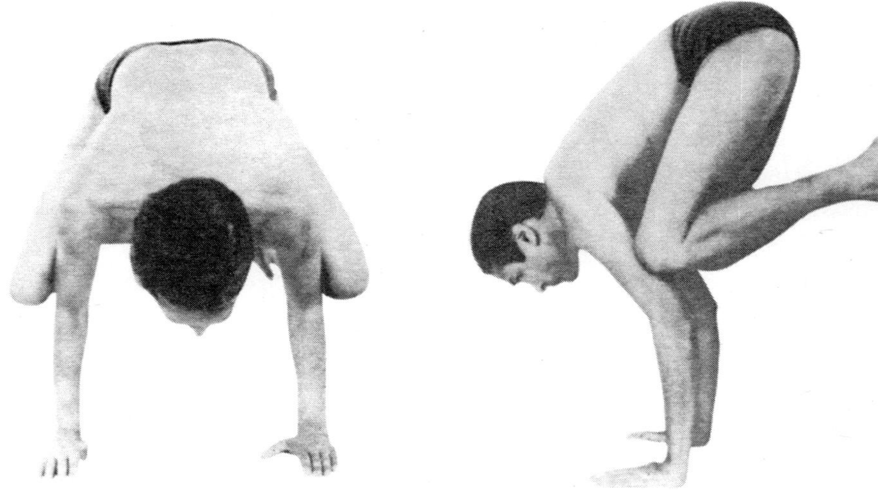

UTTHITA PADMASANA

Raised Lotus Posture

This posture strengthens the abdominal muscles, arms, wrists and hands.

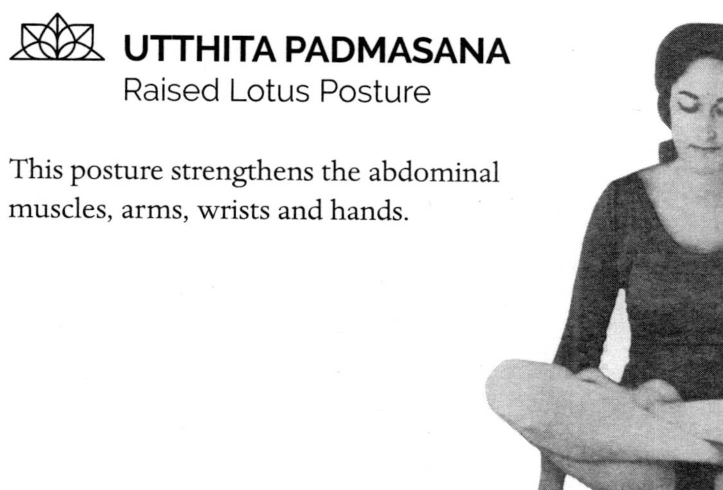

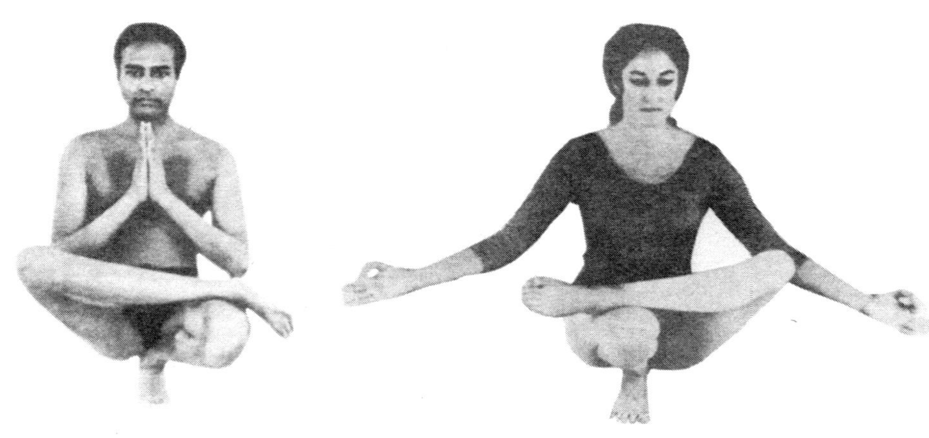

EKAPADA ANGUSHTASANA
Tiptoe Posture

This Asana fortifies the legs, ankles and feet.

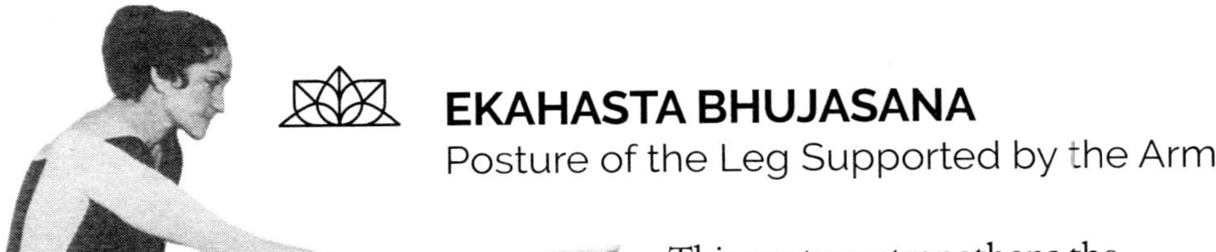

EKAHASTA BHUJASANA
Posture of the Leg Supported by the Arm

This posture strengthens the abdominal muscles, fortifies the arms, wrists and hands.

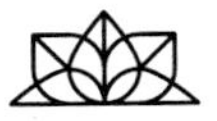

PARVATASANA
The Mountain Posture

This Asana fortifies the legs and allows the thigh and trunk muscles to be stretched to their fullest extent. It also prevents certain types of rheumatism.

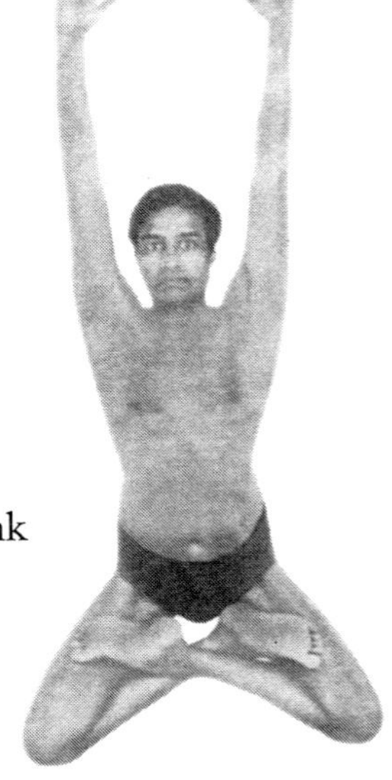

5

Asanas (Variations)

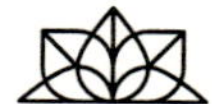

PADMASANA

Lotus Posture, Hands Joined Above Head

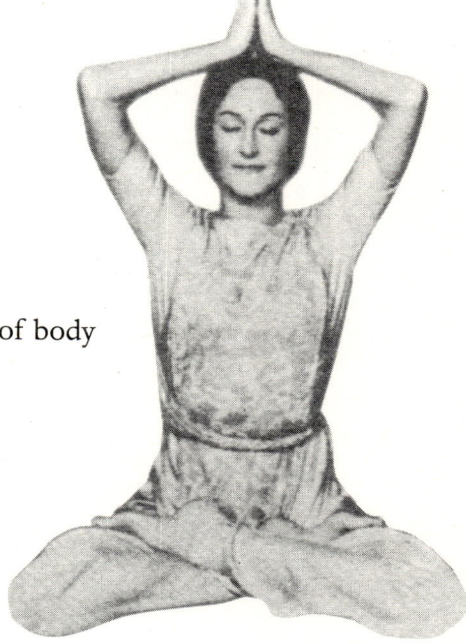

This Asana helps achieve the harmony of body and mind.

BADDHA PADMASANA
Toe-hold Lotus Posture

This posture develops the thoracic cage.

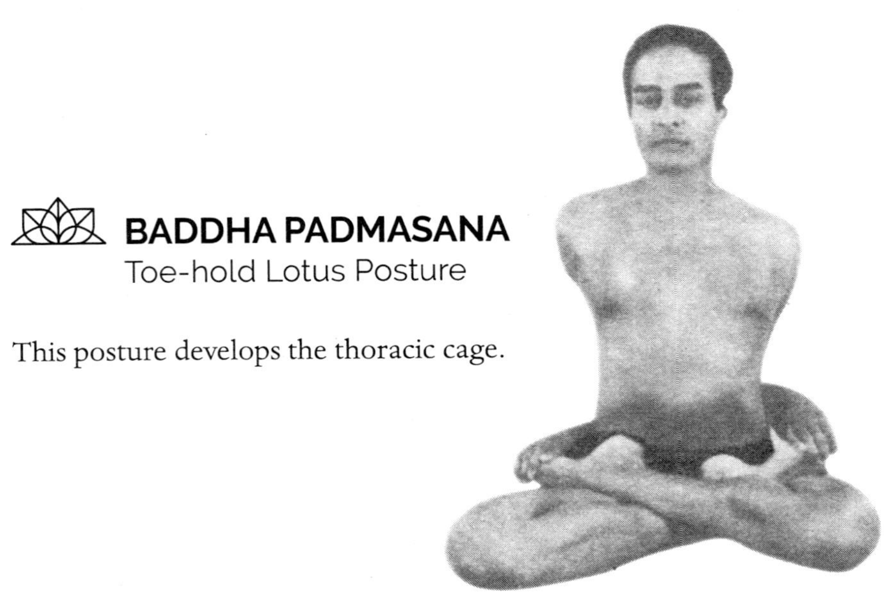

YOGA-MUDRA IN THE BADDHA PADMASANA POSITION
Toe-hold Lotus Posture, Body Leaning Forwards

This pose is effective against slow bowel movement and renders the whole body supple.

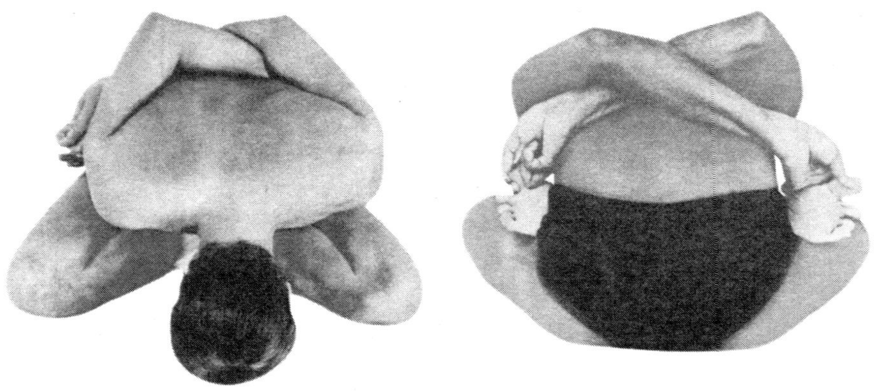

CHAKRASANA

The Wheel Posture

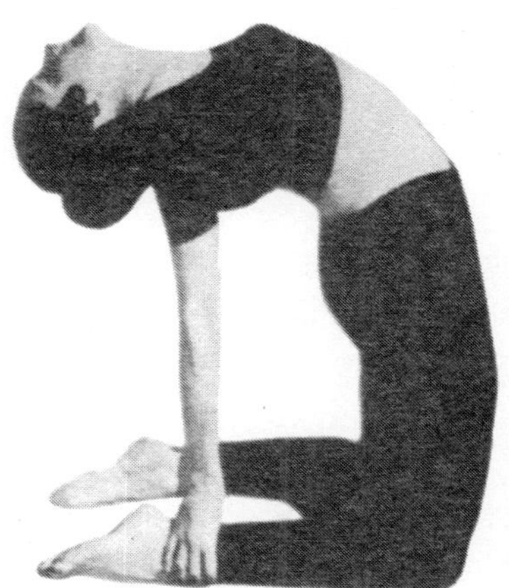

This Asana renders the spinal column flexible and develops the thoracic cage. The muscles of the abdomen, thighs and arms are strengthened, and the kidneys regenerated. It also cures infections of the trachea and larynx.

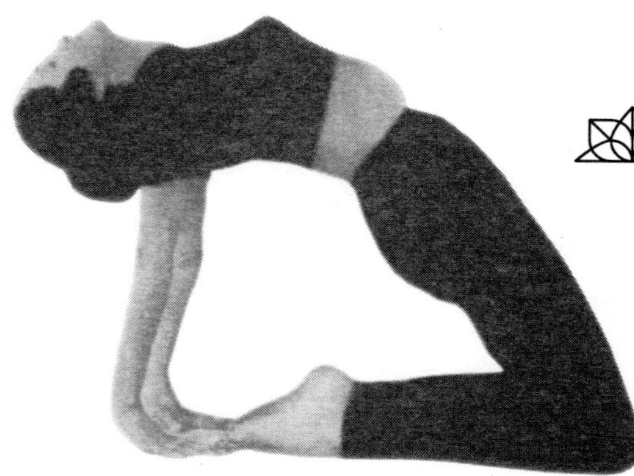

USTRASANA

The Camel Posture

The therapeutic advantages of this Asana are similar to those of Chakrasana.

MALASANA

The Garland Posture

This pose tones up the abdominal organs and soothes backaches, especially in the case of women during menstruation. It helps elongate the muscles of the back and renders the ankles more flexible.

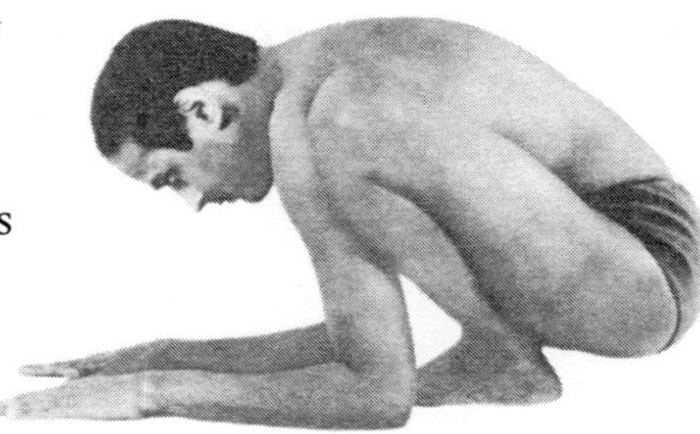

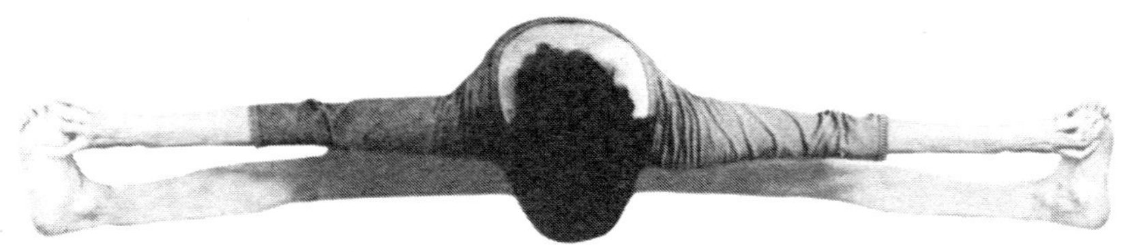

BHUNAMANASANA
Sideward Leg-stretch, Head-to-ground

This posture allows the leg muscles to be elongated, the spinal column to be stretched and the sympathetic nerve to be massaged.

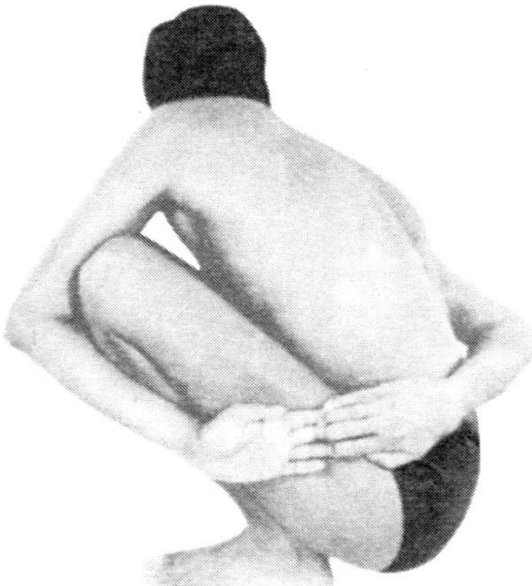

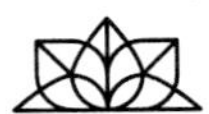

PASASANA
The Chord Posture

This Asana renders the ankles more flexible, fortifies the spinal column and gets rid of fat around the stomach. It is also beneficial to the liver, spleen and pancreas.

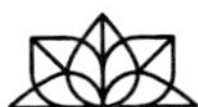

KURMASANA
The Tortoise Posture

This Asana is important to the spiritual discipline of Yoga. It develops a feeling of serenity. On a purely physical level, it has a beneficial effect on the spinal column and nervous system. The abdominal organs are also toned up by this posture. After practicing it, one feels refreshed and charged with energy.

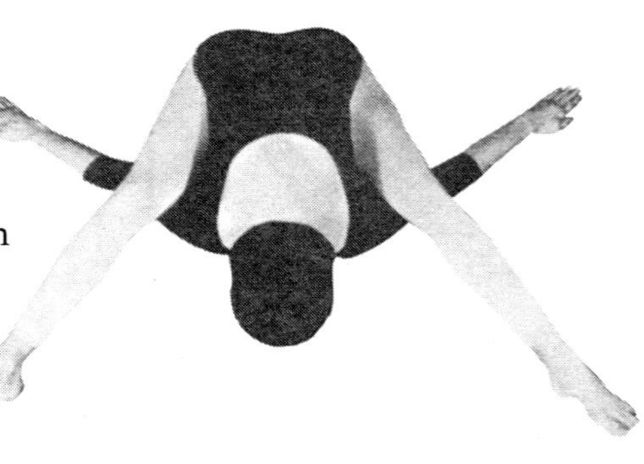

RELAXING THE BACK IN THE YOGA-MUDRA POSITION

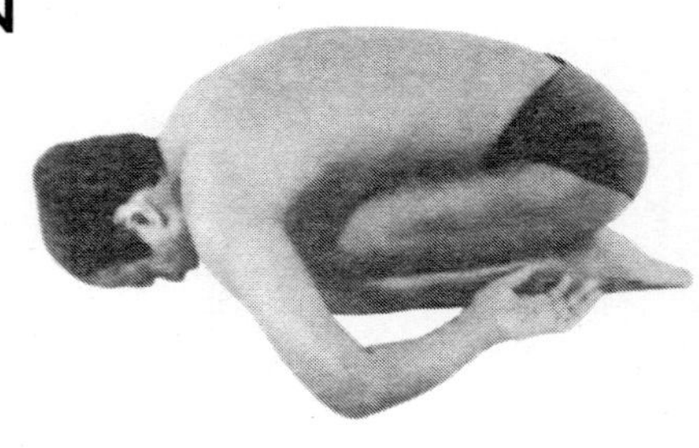

This Asana soothes backache and kidney problems. It completely relaxes the spinal column.

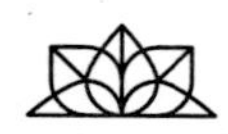

ARDHA CHANDRASANA

The Half-Moon Posture

This pose softens up the spinal column and slims down hips and waist.

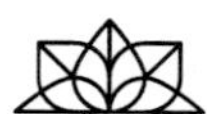

KONASANA

The Angle Posture
(standing head-to-knee)

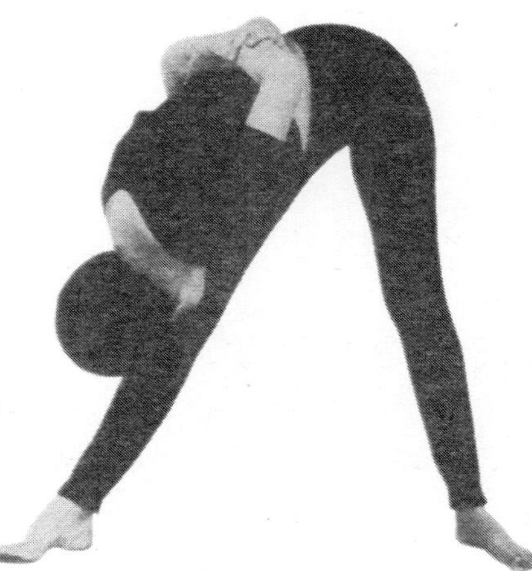

This posture renders the spinal column and hip joints more supple. All stiffness in the legs disappears, and the abdominal organs are toned up.

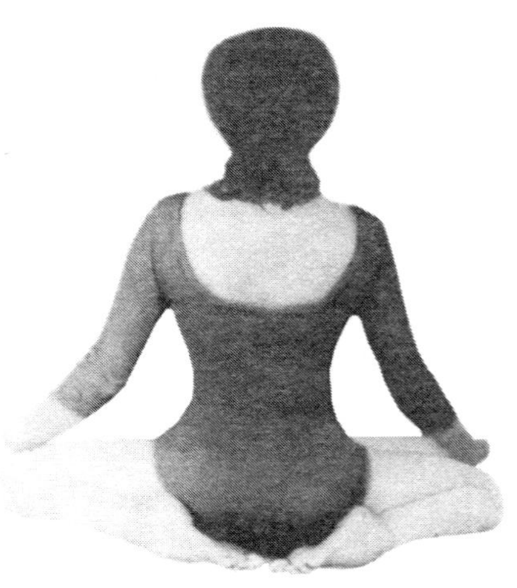

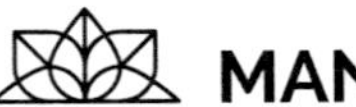

MANDUKASANA

The Frog Position

This Asana enables one to elongate the thigh muscles. When folded in this way, the legs allow a greater blood-supply to the stomach, thus helping digestion.

JANUSIRASANA

Head Touching Knee

This Asana allows the muscles of the back to be fully stretched; the legs and spinal column also become more supple. The exercise has a beneficial effect on the nervous system.

A variation of this Asana consists in placing the foot of the bent leg on the thigh of the other leg. When practiced in this way, the ankles become particularly supple.

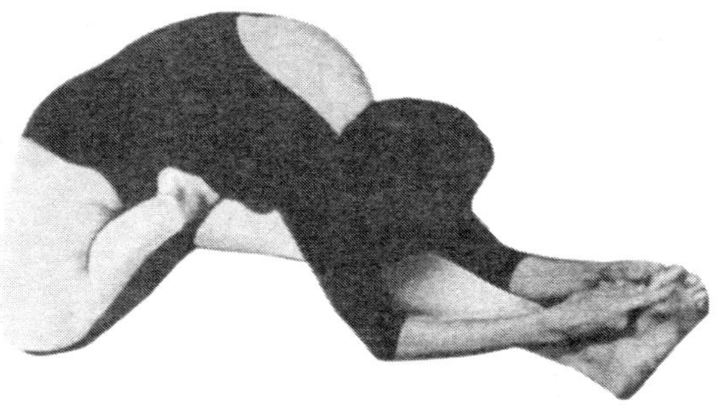

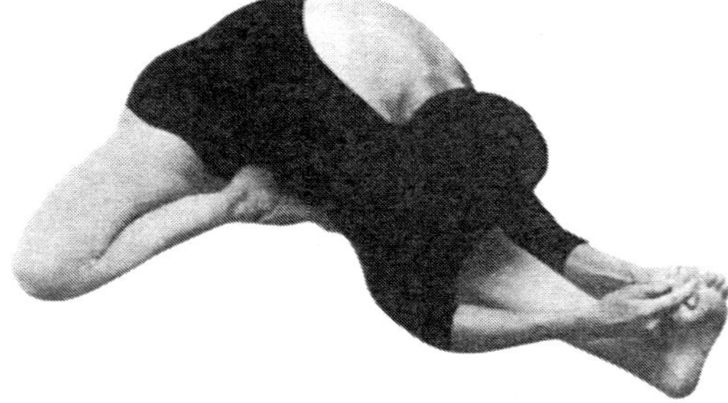

GOMUKHASANA
The Cow-Head Posture

This pose develops the arm muscles and increases the capacity of the thoracic cage.

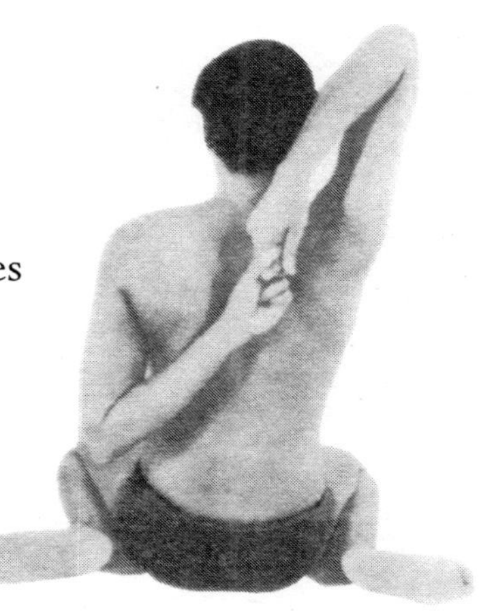

PARIVRTTA JANUSIRASANA
Head-to-knee Position, Body Leaning to One Side

This posture tones up the circulation around the spinal column. It soothes backaches and strengthens the nervous system. The legs become more supple and the exercise helps eliminate excess fat around the waist.

JANUSIRA MERUDANDASANA
Head, Knee and Spinal Column Posture

This Asana fortifies the neck and abdominal muscles maintaining the cervical and dorsal vertebrae.

PARIPURNA NAVASANA

The Boat Posture

This balancing pose strengthens the thigh and abdominal muscles. It rids the digestive organs of toxins and tones up the solar plexus. The exercise also helps develop the will-power.

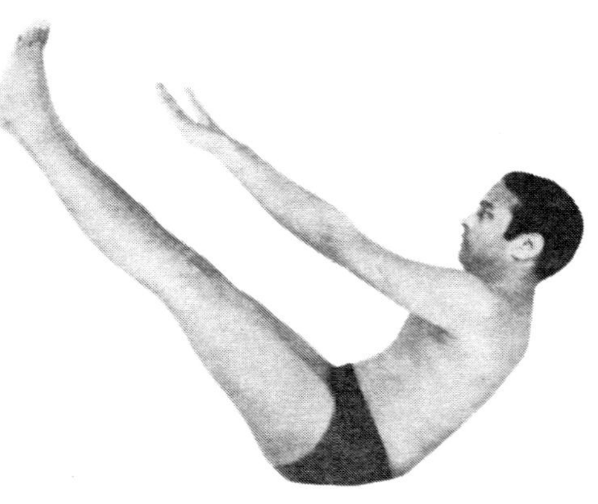

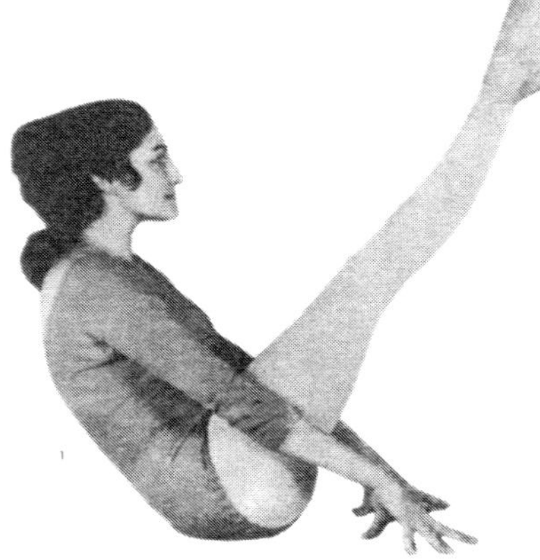

VAJROLI MUDRA

The Boat Posture, Hands on Ground

This endurance pose has therapeutic effects similar to those of Paripurna Navasana.

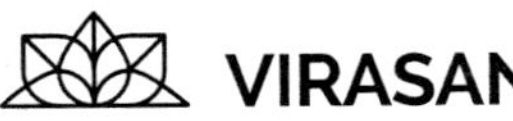

VIRASANA

The Hero Posture

This Asana is generally used for spiritual purposes. It encourages mental equilibrium and self-control.

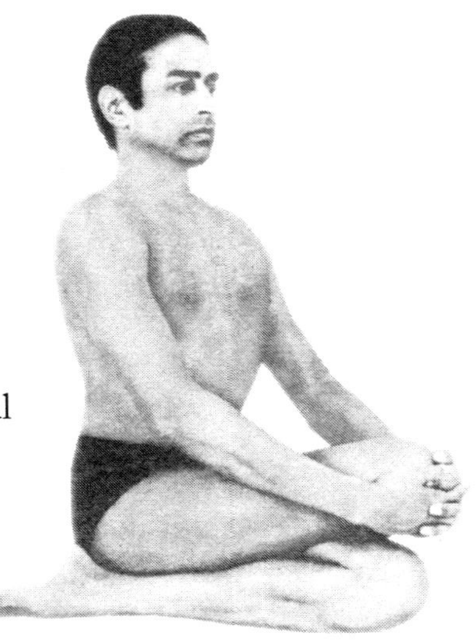

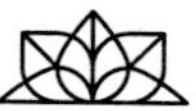

SALAMBA SIRSHASANA

Head-stand, Hands on the Ground

The therapeutic advantages of this Asana are similar to those of Sirshasana.

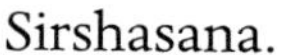

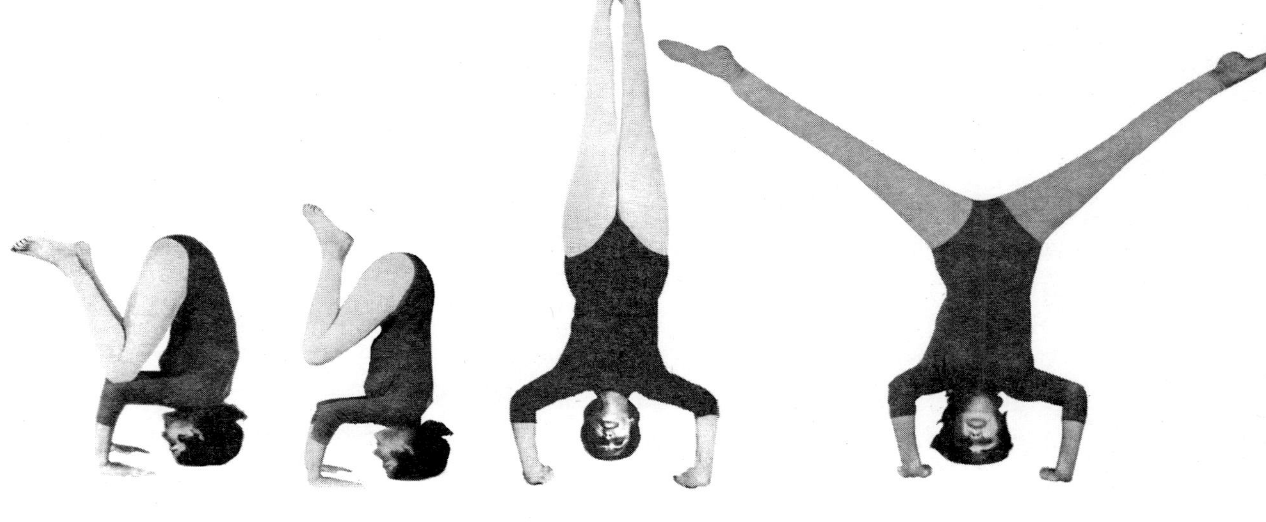

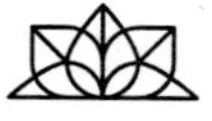

NATARAJASANA

Nataraja's Posture

This posture is dedicated to Lord Shiva, the Master of time, cosmic rhythm of life, and the source of Yoga.

In his role as cosmic dancer, Shiva is called Nataraja — the 'god of dance.'

It is a pose full of vigour and beauty, softening the body and developing the sense of equilibrium.

HOW TO KEEP THE EYES IN GOOD HEALTH

Ancient Yogic scriptures have often reiterated the fact that the eyes are sensory organs which normally function without effort and that what we see is the mind's interpretation of an image received by the retina. It has been noted that if the mind is in a highly tense state, e.g., when one is afraid or under great stress, a special effort is required to see, proving that vision is affected. This also confirms that the faculty of sight is mainly dependent upon the mind.

According to Yoga, man possesses two kinds of eyes: the external and the internal. The external eyes see the world outside, and the internal eye looks into the inner recesses of the body, helping to understand invisible forces. It is known as the 'third' eye.

The external eyes, when functioning normally, see without the slightest effort. The image received by them is transmitted to the visual centre of the brain, situated at the back of the skull, where the mind interprets it. Hence vision is a process of mental interpretation. It depends on five factors: the objects seen, the organs of sight, the sensory function, the interpretation by the brain, and the attention of the interior spirit. The mind is able to imagine objects already seen, but it cannot see them for the first time without the use of the eyes.

The interior eye or the third eye is situated between the eyebrows (Ajna Chakra). In the case of most human beings, the third eye remains dormant, but it can be awakened and developed by the will-power and the practice of Yoga. The function of the interior eye is to see invisible things, i.e., the actions and reactions of nature's forces. It is the interior eye that allows us to gain a true knowledge of a thing, action or thought. When the interior eye is awoken, the intuition develops — an extremely useful faculty to man on a physical, mental and spiritual level, in his search for perfection.

As stated above, vision, when applied to the outside world, is a complex process requiring perfect co-ordination with the mind. Yogic experiments have shown that complete relaxation with the eyes closed is very soothing to the mind and over-stressed eyes. Anyone with tired eyes may try it, all one has to do is simply close them and relax. The eyes will become relaxed and the vision sharpened.

According to Hatha-Yoga, there are three reasons why the eyes may not be functioning properly: improper use, non-use and over-use.

IMPROPER USE

It has been noted that people do not pay enough attention to the way they read or write. Few know the correct distance at which to hold a book when reading. Not only this, but they do not even blink once while reading a whole page. This is how the eyes become fatigued and painful migraines appear.

When reading, one should blink at least for every line, and when looking at a distant object, one should move the eye from one point to another while blinking.

BLINKING

One should make it a principle to hold the book at such a distance that the letters appear clearly without requiring any effort to see them. For young people, the normal distance is ten to twelve inches, and one should not forget to blink five to ten times a minute. Blinking and winking should not be confused. In blinking the upper eyelid is gently lowered and raised — a relaxing movement — while in winking, the upper eyelid touches the lower — a tiring movement. Correction of these two habits enables one to read for hours on end without the slightest discomfort.

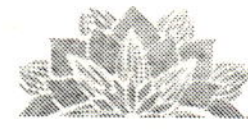

It has also been noted that some people possess certain habits when it comes to writing. As they write they simultaneously try to read what they have already written; this is a poor way of using the eyes and is also extremely tiring. What one should do is to follow the motion of the pen. To rid oneself of the habit of reading what one has just written, the latter may be hidden under a piece of paper.

Another habit is to consciously or unconsciously stare at certain objects without blinking or even moving the eyes. The proper way to look at an object is to move the eyes gently and blink lightly to avoid too much strain.

NON-USE

Experience has shown that by staying in a darkened room for a certain time, the eyes become very sensitive to bright light. It has also been observed that very many people do not use their eyes normally. They may continue in this way through negligence, or unawareness, until they realize what is happening. By relaxing the mind and eyes, the latter will soon be ready to function almost normally.

OVER-USE

Reading for hours and hours without a break is extremely taxing on the eyes; some people are even incapable of focusing on distant objects for some time afterwards. Such people should open their eyes wide and regulate their focus. This method of reading is one of the ways in which short-sightedness develops. Over-use is staring too long at near or distant objects without relaxing or blinking.

RELAXING THE EYES

Gently close the eyes and lightly cover them with the palms of the hands, resting the elbows on the knees. Let the heat from the palms penetrate the eyeballs. Make sure that the eyes are well covered and protected from all sources of light. To attain the desired results, the head should not lean backwards. The neck and spinal column should be in an upright position, but relaxed and comfortable so that neither the nerves nor muscles are strained. While inhaling and exhaling as in complete Yogic breathing, relax and let the eyes go, as if they were about to drop out. Stay in this position for a while, then lightly massage the closed eyes with the warm palms. Gently open the eyes. The soothing effects will be felt at once, and vision will be sharp and clear. From ancient times in India, the Yogis have always resorted to the palms of the hands to increase magnetic forces, for there are many nervous centres in them and they therefore possess great powers of healing.

EYE EXERCISES

The following exercises may be practised, either in the Viparitakarani (inverted) posture, the Padmasana (lotus) position, or sitting cross-legged.

TECHNIQUE

First exercise: adopt the inverted or lotus position, and after a few seconds look straight ahead. Then inhale while turning the eyes as far right as possible, and bring them back to their starting position while exhaling. Repeat, this time turning the eyes to the left. Inhale again and raise the eyes upwards, then bring them back to the original position while exhaling. Repeat, this time looking downwards.

Do not repeat more than two or three times. Stop at the first sign of strain and relax.

Second exercise: this consists in rolling the eyes in a circle. During inhalation the eyes are turned to the right, then upwards, and during exhalation they move to the left then downwards. Repeat in the reverse order. This exercise should not be performed more than two or three times. Stop at the first sign of fatigue.

Third exercise: look straight ahead. Inhale and open the eyes as wide as possible.

Exhale and clench the eyelids together for a moment. Repeat two or three times and relax.

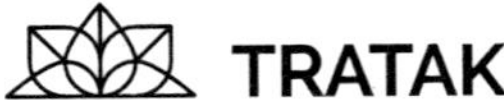

TRATAK

Exercise to increase sharp-sightedness

Tratak signifies 'central fixation' in Sanskrit. This exercise is practised to perfect the sight and improve defective vision. The black spot of the retina is the most sensitive part, for it is through this that the eye sees best. The practice of Tratak or central fixation not only develops the sensitivity of this point, but increases sharp-sightedness and improves the circulation.

TECHNIQUE

Make a white disc, six inches in diameter, and mark five black dots on it as indicated in the illustration. Place it at a distance of one to three feet.

1. Look at the black dot in the middle for a while, but without straining. Repeat this exercise two to three times.

2. First look at the black dot in the middle for a few seconds, then move the gaze over to the right dot. Return to the middle for a few seconds. Move the gaze to the left dot, return to the middle for a moment, then look at the top dot, then pass down to the bottom dot. Be sure to move the head at the same time and blink slightly. Repeat the exercise two or three times.

1. Breathe regularly and raise the eyes towards a point between the eyebrows (Bhru-madhya-drishti). Stop at the slightest sign of fatigue and relax. Do not repeat this exercise more than two or three times.

2. Breathe regularly and fix the eyes on the tip of the nose (Nasagra drishti). Relax after a few seconds. Do not repeat the exercise more than two or three times.

THERAPEUTIC ADVANTAGES

These are very good exercises for strengthening the sight. They allow one to remain sharp-sighted well into old-age.

N.B. The last two exercises, Bhru-madhya-drishti (looking towards a point between the eyebrows) and Nasagra-drishti (looking at the tip of the nose), are highly recommended for developing the powers of concentration. They should only be practised under proper guidance.

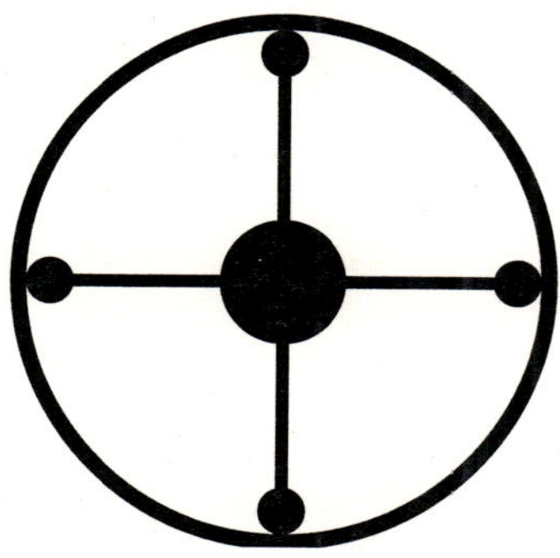

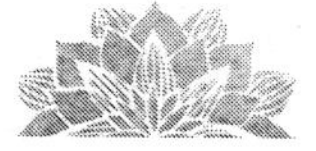

Section 3

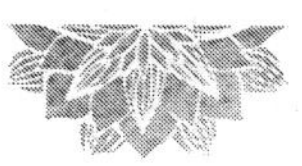

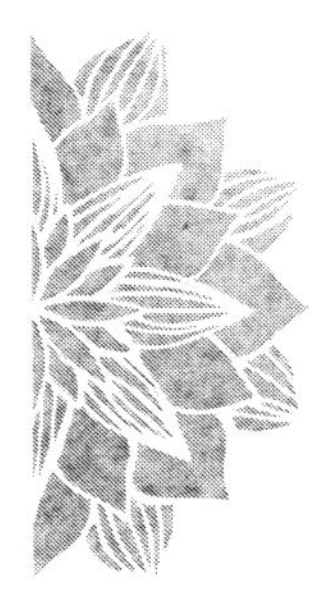

Yoga teaches us
to cure what need
not be endured
and endure what
cannot be cured.

B.K.S. Iyengar,
Founder of
Iyengar Yoga

6

The Curative Value of Pranayama and the Asanas

Most of our ills come from the weakness of the body.

— *Swami Vivekananda*

Below is a short list of various Pranayama and Asana exercises corresponding to different disorders and illnesses, both functional and organic. It is absolutely essential to ensure the guidance of a properly trained and experienced guru, who is able to adapt these exercises to the needs of the individual.

ACIDITY

Pranayama

Bhastrika (Bellows).

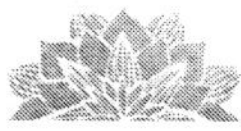

Asanas

Uddiyana (Raising of the diaphragm), Paschimottanasana (Stretching of the back and legs), Vakrasana (Spinal Twist), Mayurasana (The Peacock Posture), Trikonasana (Triangle Posture), Viparitakarani (The Inverted Posture), Savasana (Complete Relaxation Posture).

ALLERGY

Pranayama

Rhythmic breathing, Nadi-Sodhana (alternate breathing).

Asanas

Yoga-Mudra (The symbol of Yoga), Uddiyana (Raising of the diaphragm), Ardha Matsyendrasana (Simplified version of the Yogi Matsyendra Posture), Sarvangasana (Shoulder-stand), Matsyasana (The Fish Posture), Savasana (Complete Relaxation Posture).

ANEMIA

Pranayama

Ujjayi (energy-renewing Pranayama), Nadi-Sodhana (alternate breathing).

Asanas

Paschimottanasana (Stretching the back and legs), Ardha-Matsyendrasana (Simplified version of the Yogi Matsyendra Posture), Sarvangasana (Shoulder-stand), Sirshasana (Head-stand), Savasana (Complete Relaxation Posture).

ARTHRITIS

Pranayama

Rhythmic Breathing, Nadi-Sodhana (alternate breathing).

Asanas

Trikonasana (Triangle Posture). Padmasana (The Lotus Position), Salabhasana (The Locust Posture), Dhanurasana (The Bow Posture), Vakrasana (Spinal Twist), Viparitakarani (The Inverted Posture), Savasana (Complete Relaxation Posture).

ASTHMA

Pranayama

Rhythmic Breathing, Nadi-Sodhana (alternate breathing, without retention of the breath).

Asanas

Vakrasana (Spinal Twist), Paschimottanasana (Stretching the back and legs), Viparitakarani (The Inverted Posture), Savasana (Complete Relaxation Posture).

BLADDER COMPLAINTS

Pranayama

Rhythmic breathing, Nadi-Sodhana (alternate breathing).

Asanas

Uddiyana (Raising of the diaphragm), Baddhakonasana (Yoga-Mudra, feet joined), Mula-Bandha (Contraction of the pelvic and anal muscles), Paschimottanasana (Stretching the back and legs), Viparitakarani (The Inverted Posture), Savasana (Complete Relaxation Posture).

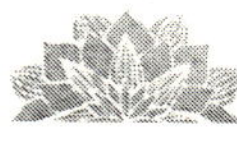

COLDS

Pranayama

Nose bath, rhythmic breathing.

Asanas

Viparitakarani (The Inverted Posture), Sarvangasana (Shoulder-stand), Savasana (Complete Relaxation Posture).

CONSTIPATION

Pranayama

Bhastrika (Bellows).

Asanas

Uddiyana (Rising of the diaphragm), Trikonasana (Triangle Posture), Vakrasana (Spinal Twist), Paschimottanasana (Stretching the back and legs), Sarvangasana (Shoulder-stand), Nauli (Isolation of the rectal and abdominal muscles), Sirshasana (Head-stand), Supta-Vajrasana (The Supine Pelvic Posture).

DIABETES

Pranayama

Rhythmic breathing, Nadi-Sodhana (alternate breathing with retention of the breath).

Asanas

Uddiyana (Raising of the diaphragm), Paschimottanasana (Stretching the back and legs), Ardha-Matsyendrasana (Simplified version of the Yogi Matsyendra Posture), Sarvangasana (Shoulder-stand), Savasana (Complete Relaxation Posture).

DIARRHOEA

Pranayama

Nadi-Sodhana (alternate breathing without retention of the breath).

Asanas

Viparitakarani (The Inverted Posture), Savasana (Complete Relaxation Posture).

EXHAUSTION

Pranayama

Rhythmic breathing, Nadi-Sodhana (alternate breathing).

Asanas

Halasana (The Plough Posture), Vakrasana (Spinal Twist), Paschimottanasana (Stretching the back and legs), Sarvangasana (Shoulder-stand), Matsyasana (The Fish Pasture), Sirshasana (Head-stand), Savasana (Complete Relaxation Posture).

HAEMORROIDS

Pranayama

Rhythmic breathing, Breathing that revitalizes the nervous system.

Asanas

Uddiyana (Raising of the diaphragm), Viparitakarani (The Inverted Posture), Sarvangasana (Shoulder-stand), Matsyasana (The Fish Posture), Sirshasana (Head-stand), Savasana (Complete Relaxation Posture).

HEADACHES

Pranayama

Rhythmic breathing, Nadi-Sodhana (alternate breathing).

Asanas

Viparitakarani (The Inverted Posture), Savasana (Complete Relaxation Posture).

HEART TROUBLE

Pranayama

Rhythmic breathing, Nadi-Sodhana (alternate breathing without retention of the breath).

Asanas (Depending on the case)

Uddiyana (Raising of the diaphragm), Trikonasana (Triangle Posture), Sirshasana (Head-stand), Savasana (Complete Relaxation Posture).

HERNIA

Pranayama

Rhythmic breathing, Nadi-Sodhana (alternate breathing).

Asanas

Baddha-Konasana (Yoga-Mudra. feet joined), Uddiyana (Raising of the diaphragm), Sarvangasana (Shoulder-stand), Savasana (Complete Relaxation Posture).

HIGH BLOOD PRESSURE

Pranayama

Rhythmic breathing, Nadi-Sodhana (alternate breathing, without retention of the breath).

Asanas

Padmasana (The Lotus Position), Viparitakarani (The Inverted Posture), Savasana (Complete Relaxation Posture).

IMPOTENCY

Pranayama

Rhythmic breathing, Kumbhaka (retention of the breath), Nadi-Sodhana (alternate breathing).

Asanas

Yoga-Mudra (The Symbol of Yoga), Uddiyana (Raising of the diaphragm), Mula-Bandha (Contraction of the pelvic and anal muscles), Dhanurasana (The Bow Posture), Ardha-Matsyendrasana (Simplified version of the Yogi Matsyendra Posture), Paschimottanasana (Stretching the back and legs), Sarvangasana (Shoulder-stand), Matsyasana (The Fish Posture), Sirshasana (Head-stand), Savasana (Complete Relaxation Posture).

INDIGESTION

Pranayama

Bhastrika (Bellows), Nadi-Sodhana (alternate breathing).

Asanas

Uddiyana (Raising of the diaphragm), Bhujangasana (The Cobra Position), Salabhasana (The Locust Posture), Dhanurasana (The Bow Posture), Trikonasana (Triangle Posture), Paschimottanasana (Stretching the back and legs), Sarvangasana (Shoulder-stand), Savasana (Complete Relaxation Posture).

KIDNEY COMPLAINTS

Pranayama

Rhythmic breathing, Nadi-Sodhana (alternate breathing).

Asanas

Yoga-Mudra (The Symbol of Yoga), Uddiyana (Raising of the diaphragm), Bhujangasana (The Cobra Posture). Salabhasana (The Locust Posture), Dhanurasana (The Bow Posture), Vakrasana (Spinal Twist), Paschimottanasana (Stretching the back and legs), Sarvangasana (Shoulder-stand), Savasana (Complete Relaxation Posture).

LIVER AILMENTS

Pranayama

Rhythmic breathing, Nadi-Sodhana (alternate breathing).

Asanas

Uddiyana (Raising of the diaphragm), Baddha-Konasana (Yoga-Mudra, feet joined), Mayurasana (The Peacock Posture), Paschimottanasana (Stretching the back and legs). Viparitakarani (The Inverted Posture), Savasana (Complete Relaxation Posture).

LOW BLOOD PRESSURE

Pranayama

Rhythmic breathing, Bhastrika (Bellows).

Asanas

Siddhasana (Posture of the Adept), Halasana (The Plough Posture), Paschimottanasana (Stretching the back and legs), Sarvangasana (Shoulder-stand), Sirshasana (Head-stand), Savasana (Complete Relaxation Posture).

OBESITY OR OVERWEIGHT

Pranayama

Bhastrika (Bellows), Ujjayi (energy-renewing Pranayama), Kapalabhati (breathing that revitalizes the body).

Asanas

Uddiyana (Raising of the diaphragm), Paschimottanasana (Stretching the back and legs), Trikonasana (Triangle Posture), Vakrasana (Spinal Twist), Sarvangasana (Shoulder-stand), Sirshasana (Head-stand), Dhanurasana (The Bow Posture).

PARALYSIS

Pranayama

Rhythmic breathing, Nadi-Sodhana (alternate breathing), Ujjayi (energy-renewing Pranayama).

Asanas *(depending on the case)*

Bhujangasana (The Cobra Posture), Salabhasana (The Locust Posture), Dhanurasana (The Bow Posture), Halasana (The Plough Posture), Viparitakarani (The Inverted Posture), Savasana (Complete Relaxation Posture).

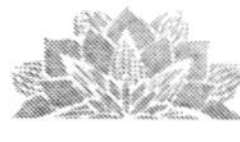

RHEUMATISM

Pranayama

Rhythmic breathing, Nadi-Sodhana (alternate breathing).

Asanas

Trikonasana (Triangle Posture), Bhujangasana (The Cobra Posture), Salabhasana (The Locust Posture), Dhanurasana (The Bow Posture), Ardha-Matsyendrasana (Simplified version of the Yogi Matsyendra Posture), Sarvangasana (Shoulder-stand), Savasana (Complete Relaxation Posture).

SINUS TROUBLE

Pranayama

Nadi-Sodhana (alternate breathing), Surya Bhedana.

Asanas

Viparitakarani (The Inverted Posture), Savasana (Complete Relaxation Posture).

STERILITY

Pranayama

Rhythmic breathing, Nadi-Sodhana (alternate breathing), Ujjayi (energy-renewing Pranayama).

Asanas

Yoga-Mudra (The Symbol of Yoga), Supta-Vajrasana (The Supine Pelvic Posture), Mula-Bandha (Contraction of the pelvic and anal muscles), Paschimottanasana (Stretching the back and legs), Vakrasana (Spinal Twist), Sarvangasana (Shoulder-stand), Sirshasana (Head-stand), Dhanurasana (The Bow Posture).

TUBERCULOSIS

(in its early stages)

Pranayama

Rhythmic breathing, Nadi-Sodhana (alternate breathing).

Asanas

Viparitakarani (The Inverted Posture), Sarvangasana (Shoulder-stand), Sirshasana (Head-stand), Savasana (Complete Relaxation Posture).

ULCER

(beginnings of)

Pranayama

Rhythmic breathing, Ujjayi (energy-renewing Pranayama), Nadi-Sodhana (alternate breathing).

Asanas

Uddiyana (Raising of the diaphragm), Paschimottanasana (Stretching the back and legs), Ardha-Matsyendrasana (Simplified version of the Yogi Matsyendra Posture), Sarvangasana (Shoulder-stand), Sirshasana (Head-stand), Savasana (Complete Relaxation Posture).

VARICOSE VEINS

Pranayama

Nadi-Sodhana (alternate breathing), Bhastrika (Bellows).

Asanas

Padmasana (The Lotus Position), Yoga-Mudra (The Symbol of Yoga), Vakrasana (Spinal Twist), Viparitakarani (The Inverted Posture), Sarvangasana (Shoulder-stand), Matsyasana (The Fish Posture), Sirshasana (Head-stand), Savasana (Complete Relaxation Posture).

7

Yogic Therapy for Various Illnesses of Psychic Origin

> Our personal development is influenced by each of our thoughts and deeds.
>
> — *Dhammapada*

All humans have a body, mind and soul. The mind is the seat of the instincts and the emotional life, while the soul is the Self, the divine spark that is part of our consciousness. The body is the temple of the soul and the instrument by which the Self is made manifest. It is therefore of crucial importance to preserve the body in perfect health.

To be in good health we should begin by the inner consciousness; this is only possible, however, by means of the mental processes. If we want to be healthy in body, our emotions have to be in unison with the life-force inside each one of us.

We need to realize that every negative mental or emotional state is destructive, while a positive one tends to heal the body and assist in preservation of a healthy state. Behind every illness there is a state of mental disorder, for the body is the projection of the consciousness; thoughts, sentiments, beliefs and attitudes have a direct influence on our health. A negative thought, sentiment or word is like a command to the subconscious mind for an illness.

Whenever we control our mental and emotional attitude, transforming it from a negative to a positive one, we are able to remedy unfavourable physical conditions. When, for example, we can dominate our fears and transform them into confidence, we are full of hope, dynamism and self-assurance. Similarly worry may be brought under control and transformed into serenity; jealousy turned into benevolence; stress into relaxation; hostility into love and incomprehension into understanding; agitation into tranquility; selfishness into selflessness; greed into generosity; condemnation into tolerance; nervousness into calm; frustration into expression; sadness into joy, and so on... all of which help us obtain a state of perfect health and inner happiness.

The close relationship between our mental attitude, emotional attitude and our general state of health is of critical importance. In recent years, medical science has also validated that the mental and physical states are very closely connected. Most people do not, however, relate the state of their mind to the condition of their body.

I should like to make the reader fully aware of such facts, and help him develop those attitudes and mental states which will free the inner forces of nature, ensuring good health and happiness. He should realize that a person can only recover from sickness when he changes his state of mind. *The effects will only disappear once the cause has been eliminated*. Surgeons and doctors are able to save lives and relieve pain, but the patient can only be healed if his inner consciousness co-operates with the natural life-force which flows within him.

The Remarkable Power of Positive Auto-Suggestion

In many instances, sickness can be cured by the simple use of positive auto-suggestion. We tire ourselves out by feeling tense; we become nervous, irritable, and can even fall sick. Uncontrolled thoughts and emotions are a factor causing imbalance, which may be the origin of disorders in the body. It is obvious, therefore, that to find a cure, the latent cause has to be treated, even though it may often be hidden by the sickness. Unfortunately, the ignorance or scepticism of many patients makes them incapable of using this remarkable power of positive auto-suggestion; their materialistic outlook and inability to acknowledge this kind of healing, even their aversion to it, deprives them of the help this therapeutic aid has to offer.

Faith is another essential aspect of the healing process. I am able to cite many cases of patients who were cured by the sheer power of faith. 'It cannot be denied that such miracles and answers to people's prayers result from the power of conviction and affirmative suggestion, which goes to show that man is a receptacle for the infinite ocean of power that lies within himself' (Swami Vivekananda). The tangible reality behind this phenomenon is that the force of affirmative suggestion and the power of faith are so intense that they penetrate into the inner consciousness of the individual producing an immediate reaction and bringing the desired results. All those who, in the course of centuries, have devoted themselves to the cultivation of the powers of the mind are correct in regarding mental force, when directed positively, as a highly efficient method for treating sickness, even in the case of those who do not respond to traditional therapy.

The same is also true where the sickness does not have any apparent mental origin, but is due to a virus or infection, or demands immediate surgery. Even in cases as these, the patient will get better very quickly if his moral and mental attitude remain positive and optimistic.

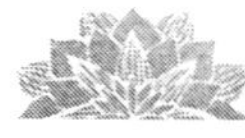

Even recently, it was still believed that sickness had a purely physical origin. Progress in psychoanalysis has shown that most physical illnesses are the result of emotional or mental disturbance. This discovery is now known as 'psychosomatic medicine'.

The Greek word 'Psyche' means 'soul', and 'Soma' 'body'. Several clinics specializing in psychosomatic medicine have recently confirmed that emotional tension, when unable to find expression in words or actions, takes the form of an illness.

> If the mind is the source of all physical ills of psychic and emotional origin, it may also be the source of healing.

The truth of this was already known in India, where Yoga existed, several thousand years ago.

It has been observed, in the light of Yogic experience, that if the mind dominates the emotions and the consciousness develops equally in the various directions required, then energy will be uniformly spread throughout the various nervous and mental centres. The body will thus be kept in perfect health, for the positive and negative currents, i.e., life-giving and life-receiving, that keep it alive, will be in perfect equilibrium.

Vital energy is constantly active within us, bringing us equilibrium, and as long as we live naturally, keeping us in good health. Sickness is nothing more than an unnatural way of life and unbaianced mind. Regular practice of Yoga, i.e., the Asanas, Pranayama, and mental discipline, will teach us how to use, store and maximise the free circulation of vital energy within the body.

As soon as one of the two kinds of energy, either positive or negative is directed in one direction only, whether to the mind or to the body, we open the doors to many disorders. It has been observed that in general, those who concentrate on incessant intellectual work, to the neglect of the body, are often physically extremely weak and hence have low resistance. Those who work constantly on the physical level, however, often have rather dull minds. This goes to show that an individual's equilibrium is disturbed when his consciouness is thrown out of balance.

If a person uses his force of mind in the wrong direction, his body will sooner or later fall ill. On account of negative attitude, such a person doubts everything — has confidence neither in himself, nor in others. He is afraid of everything and sees evil in everything; thus he wrecks his life, while at the same time looking for help in every direction. This proves that the negative force of mind completely neutralizes the positive energy. *One should never, therefore, be negative in thoughts, words and in actions. All passive or negative attitudes to life must necessarily be transformed into positive ones that are dynamic, favouring all our activities.*

Let us take an example: Insomnia.

This is without doubt the most common and widely spread complaint of today. Barbiturates, tranquillizers and sleeping pills — even when taken under medical supervision — do not produce satisfactory results. On the contrary: they act as depressants, not only on the respiratory system, but also on the entire nervous system. Those who become addicted use them regularly and are tempted to take more and more. They often pass the limits because they do not bear in mind the doses they have already swallowed, and continue to imagine that they will not be able to sleep. Generally speaking, they feel giddy, often have convulsions and even delirium, while some fall into a kind of coma.

In short, barbiturates, tranquillizers and sleeping pills are not only dangerous for the nervous system, but often fatal.

Medical reports and psychosomatic medicine agree with Yogic research. They confirm that there are several underlying psychic causes for every human problem. In the case of insomnia, for

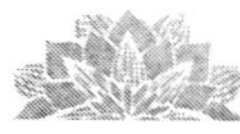

example, a large number of people have come to me hoping that Yoga would help them. Analysis of their cases has always shown that there was a dread of something quite specific buried in their subconscious mind. Once this fear had been removed, they immediately felt relieved, regained confidence and were able to sleep again.

We should never lose sight of the fact that the human mind is capable of imagining all sorts of spectres originating from anxiety, a fundamental factor in all human problems. Life is completely poisoned and destroyed by it.

It is of the greatest importance, therefore, that we eliminate all specific dread and transform it into a positive outlook. Apart from fear itself, *there are other psychic causes of insomnia*, e.g., tension, guilt-complexes, mental disorientation, anxiety, inability to face up to the responsibilities of life. *Positive attitudes which should be adopted*: relaxation, equilibrium, order, confidence, faith.

Pranayama: rhythmic breathing, Nadi-Sodhana (alternate breathing), Kumbhaka (retention of the breath). *Asanas*: Paschimottansana (Stretching of the back and legs), Viparitakarani (The Inverted Posture), Ardha-Matsyendrasana (Simplified version of the Yogi Matsyendra Posture), Trikonasana (Triangle Posture), Savasana (Complete Relaxation Posture).

Experience of Yoga shows us that regular practice of the Asanas and suitable Pranayama exercises plus the harmonious disposition of the consciousness, help us to quickly develop tendencies of positive mental approach.

There are numerous examples of physical and psychic improvements going hand-in-hand — for it has been proved that as soon as the process of mental adjustment has been accomplished, the physical state changes for the better. From the moment patient's attitude to life and his fellow men is transformed within his inner consciousness, he is on the road to recovery.

Hence we may conclude that *the power of positive thought, when directed to the inner consciousness of the patient, is capable of producing the desired results.*

Modern drugs are able to produce temporary relief, so that the patient's condition improves momentarily. As long as the patient's mental attitude remains negative, however, he will make no progress in developing the moral force required to overcome difficulties; hence improvement will not be permanent. *The surest way to combat the causes of various illnesses of psychic origin is through the positive process of affirmations within oneself.*

We will never be able to have a body that is full of vitality, nor maintain ourselves in a positive mental and emotional state, unless we follow the laws of interior harmony.

To preserve perfect health, we must know how to breathe properly, relax completely, both physically and mentally, practise the Asanas and Pranayama exercises, and follow a well-balanced diet.

Since it is not possible to cover all illnesses nor go into each case in detail describing symptoms and psychic causes, I shall simply list some of the more common ones. They are meant to be taken only as examples, for their causes and effects may differ from case to case. The examples given here are aimed at drawing the reader's attention towards the origins of a particular illness and the way of eliminating them through Yoga.

ANXIETY

Causes

Tension, fear, pessimism, egocentricity.

Attitudes to be adopted

Think of others, relax, optimism, faith.

Pranayama

Kapalabhati (breathing that revives the body), Nadi-Sodhana (alternate breathing), Kumbhaka (retention of the breath).

Asanas

Supta-Vajrasana (The Supine Pelvic Posture), Ardha-Matsyendrasana (Simplified version of the Yogi Matsyendra Posture), Trikonasana (Triangle Posture), Dhanurasana (The Bow Posture), Sarvangasana (Shoulder-stand), Savasana (Complete Relaxation Posture).

DEPRESSION

Causes

Overwork, nervousness, anxiety, pessimism, feeling of unfulfilment.

Attitudes to be adopted

Rest, calm, optimism, faith, fulfilment.

Pranayama

Rhythmic breathing, Surya-Bhedana (breathing that revitalizes the nervous system), Bhastrika (Bellows).

Asanas

Vakrasana (Spinal Twist), Bhujangasana (The Cobra Posture), Salabhasana (The Locust Posture), Halasana (The Plough Posture), Paschimottanasana (Stretching the back and legs), Sarvangasana (Shoulder-stand), Savasana (Complete Relaxation Posture).

NOCTURNAL EMISSIONS

Causes

Fear and anxiety, insecurity, frustration, tension.

Attitudes to be adopted

Self-confidence, serentiy, self-fulfilment, calm.

Pranayama

Rhythmic breathing, Nadi-Sodhana (alternate breathing), Ujjayi, (energy-renewing breathing).

Assanas

Mula-Bandha (Contraction of the pelvic and anal muscles), Baddha Konasana (Yoga-Mudra, feet joined), Paschimottanasana (Stretching the back and legs), Sarvangasana (Shoulder-stand), Savasana (Complete Relaxation Posture).

FATIGUE

Causes

Useless conflicts, disorder, agitation, tension, nervousness, overwork.

Attitudes to be adopted

Appeasement, order, tranquillity, relaxation, calm.

Pranayama

Rhythmic breathing, Nadi-Sodhana (alternate breathing), Ujjayi (energy-renewing breathing).

Asanas

Halasana (The Plough Posture), Paschimottansana (Stretching the back and legs), Ardha-Matsyendrasana (Simplified version of Yogi Matsyendra Posture), Sarvangasana (Shoulder-stand), Matsyasana (The Fish Posture), Sirshasana (Head-stand), Savasana (Complete Relaxation Posture).

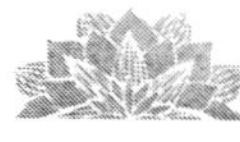

NERVOUSNESS

Causes

Disorder and lack of organization, rushing and hurrying, agitation, tension, insecurity, irrationability, anxiety.

Attitudes to be adopted

Order and organization, calm, poise, relaxation, confidence, serenity, peace.

Pranayama

Rhythmic breathing, Nadi-Sodhana (alternate breathing).

Asanas

Yoga-Mudra (The Symbol of Yoga), Vakrasana (Spinal Twist), Salabhasana (The Locust Posture), Halasana (The Plough Posture), Mayurasana (The Peacock Posture), Viparita-karani (The Inverted Posture), Savasana (Complete Relaxation Posture).

MENSTRUAL DISORDERS

Causes

Tension, anxiety, insecurity, frustration, rejection.

Attitudes to be adopted

Relaxation, faith, serenity, self-fulfilment, affirmation.

Pranayama

Rhythmic breathing, Nadi-Sodhana (alternate breathing), Kumbhaka (retention of the breath).

Asanas

Badha Konasana (Yoga-Mudra, feet joined), Vakrasana (Spinal Twist), Uddiyana (Raising of the diaphragm), Sarvangasana (Head-stand), Matsyasana (The Fish Posture), Savasana (Complete Relaxation Posture).

8

The Psychological Causes of Human Problems of Yoga

> Success is the fruit of unflagging perseverance and unshakeable will.
>
> — *Swami Vivekananda*

Every individual encounters difficulties in the course of his existence. Quite apart from physical and psychological illnesses, there are many problems in our lives. Doctors, psychologists and psychiatrists all try to solve them, but in fact, it is we ourselves who solve them by becoming conscious and co-operating with the natural forces of life within us.

Fear, hostile attitudes, inferiority and guilt complexes are the causes of psychological problems, while faith, love, confidence and tolerance are positive, constructive forces. We must therefore rid ourselves of negative mental states by certain specific affirmations, i.e., transform the negative into positive attitudes. Once we have

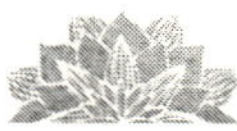

done so we would have eliminated all our problems and difficulties, thus improving our entire life by living in a state of happiness and harmony.

'Where there is a problem, there is a solution', says an ancient Hindu proverb. Whenever we have a problem, we must correct the cause, for in this way the difficulty disappears. To achieve this, absolute mental discipline is required, i.e., we should train the mind to remain totally conscious of what it is thinking, saying and doing.

This is why all ancient texts on Yoga continually repeat that disciplining of the mind is absolutely indispensable, and the practice of Asanas and Pranayama will help to achieve the required results.

To conclude, Yoga is not just a system of physical postures or breathing exercises, beneficial to health, youth and longevity — as certain people believe — but an art of living harmoniously and creatively on the basis of a complete experience of the whole being.

It is a method which aims at opening the source of creative inspiration hidden inside the human psyche. It is an act of self-manifestation and the multiplicity of our being. Yoga lays the foundations for a higher form of self-development and a deeper consciousness of self, eliminating the undesirable psychological causes of all human problems.

Three main points will help the reader become more aware of the process of self-development and eliminate various personal problems. He should:

1. Completely eliminate the negative states of consciousness.
2. Bring them into harmony by positive, constructive mental attitudes.
3. Practise the Asanas and Pranayama.

In the following pages, the reader will find a number of examples of some of the most common human problems which I have encountered in my years of teaching and thanks to Yoga discipline, have produced surprising results.

INDECISION

Causes

Timorous attitude, weakness, absent-mindedness, lack of purpose and ideals, inability to concentrate, lack of assurance, sloth and lack of initiative.

Attitudes to be adopted

Courage, firmness, will-power, aims and ideals, disciplined thought, self-confidence, initiative.

Pranayama

Rhythmic breathing, Nadi-Sodhana (alternate breathing,) Kumbhaka (retention of the breath).

Asanas

Yoga-Mudra (The Symbol of Yoga), Uddiyana (Raising of the Diaphragm), Supta-Vajrasana (The Supine Pelvic Posture), Vakrasana (Spinal Twist), Bhujangasana (The Cobra Posture), Viparitakarani (The Inverted Posture), Savasana (Complete Relaxation Posture).

HASTE

Causes

Impatience, lack of organization, disorder, nervousness.

Attitudes to be adopted

Patience, organization, order, calm.

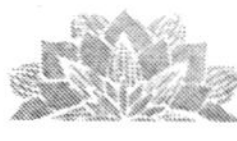

Pranayama

Rhythmic breathing, Kapalabhati (breathing that revitalizes the body), Nadi-Sodhana (alternate breathing).

Asanas

Vakrasana (Spinal Twist), Supta-Vajrasana (The Supine Pelvic Posture), Dhanurasana (The Bow Posture), Mayurasana (The Peacock Posture), Sarvangasana (Shoulder-stand), Sirshasana (Head-stand), Savasana (Complete Relaxation Posture).

NERVOUSNESS

Causes

Haste, irrationality of thought, useless conflicts, agitation.

Attitudes to be adopted

Poise, order, appeasement, calm.

Pranayama

Rhythmic breathing, Nadi-Sodhana (alternate breathing without retention of the breath).

Asanas

Paschimottanasana (Stretching of the back and leg), Viparitakarani (The Inverted Posture), Sarvangasana (Shoulder-stand), Matsyasana (The Fish Posture), Sirshasana (Head-stand) Savasana (Complete Relaxation Posture).

EXCESSIVE TOUCHINESS

Causes

Inferiority complex, lack of understanding, egocentricity, guilt complex.

Attitudes to be adopted

Peace of mind, self-confidence, understanding and tolerance, selflessness.

Pranayama

Rhythmic breathing, Bhastrika (Bellows), Nadi-Sodhana (alternate breathing).

Asanas

Uddiyana (Raising of the diaphragm), Yoga-Mudra (The Symbol of Yoga), Ardha-Matsyendrasana (Simplified version of the Yogi Matsyendra Posture), Halasana (The Plough Posture), Sarvangasana (Shoulder-stand), Savasana (Complete Relaxation Posture).

NIGHTMARES

Causes

Fear, guilt, depression and anxiety, lack of self-confidence, tension.

Attitudes to be adopted

Faith, serenity, calm and peace, self-confidence, relaxation.

Pranayama

Kapalabhati (breathing that revitalizes the body), Ujjayi (energy-renewing Pranayama), Bhastrika (Bellows).

Asanas

Uddiyana (Raising of the diaphragm), Supta-Vajrasana (The Supine Pelvic Posture), Mayurasana (The Peacock Posture), Paschimottanasana (Stretching the back and legs), Viparitakarani (The Inverted Posture), Sirshasana (Head-stand), Savasana (Complete Relaxation Posture).

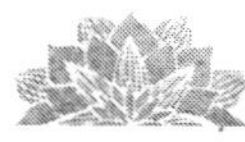

DISHARMONY

Causes

Sudden changes of mood, pettiness, hostility to others, emotional conflicts, selfishness, anxiety.

Attitudes to be adopted

Evenness of temper, tolerance and generosity, kindness, inner peace, selflessness, faith.

Pranayama

Rhythmic breathing, Kumbhaka (retention of the breath), Nadi-Sodhana (alternate breathing).

Asanas

Yoga-Mudra (The Symbol of Yoga), Vakrasana (Spinal Twist), Mayurasana (The Peacock Posture), Paschimottanasana (Stretching the back and legs), Sarvangasana (Shoulder-stand), Savasana (Complete Relaxation Posture).

OBSESSION

Causes

Mistrust, anxiety, guilt complex, fear, superstition, lack of self-confidence.

Attitudes to be adopted

Confidence, relaxation, understanding, faith.

Pranayama

Rhythmic breathing, Nadi-Sodhana (alternate breathing), Bhastrika (Bellows).

Asanas

Uddiyana (Raising of the diaphragm), Vakrasana (Spinal Twist),

Halasana (The Plough Posture), Paschimottanasana (Stretching the back and legs), Sarvangasana (Shoulder-stand), Sirshasana (Head-stand), Savasana (Complete Relaxation Posture).

MELANCHOLY

Causes

Lack of a sense of humour, fear, moroseness, negative attitudes, pessimism, depression.

Attitudes to be adopted

Sense of humour, faith, gaiety, positive attitudes, optimism, liveliness and enthusiasm.

Pranayama

Breathing that purifies, Nadi-Sodhana (alternate breathing), Bhastrika (Bellows).

Asanas

Supta-Vajrasana (The Supine Pelvic Posture), Trikonasana (Triangle Posture), Ardha-Matsyendrasana (Simplified version of the Yogi Matsyendra Posture), Halasana (The Plough Posture), Sarvangasana (Shoulder-stand), Sirshasana (Head-stand), Savasana (Complete Relaxation Posture).

FRUSTRATION

Causes

Lack of interest in life, narrow-mindedness, excessive reserve, lack of courage, inhibitions, selfishness.

Attitudes to adopt

Enthusiasm and interest in life, open-mindedness, interest in others, fulfilment, selflessness.

Pranayama

Rhythmic breathing, Nadi-Sodhana (Alternate Breathing), breathing that purifies.

Asanas

Baddha Konasana (Yoga-Mudra, feet joined), Halasana (The Plough Posture), Vakrasana (Spinal Twist), Sarvangasana (Shoulder-stand), Savasana (Complete Relaxation Posture).

Section 4

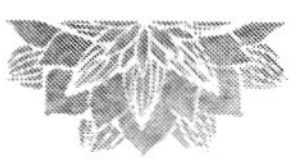

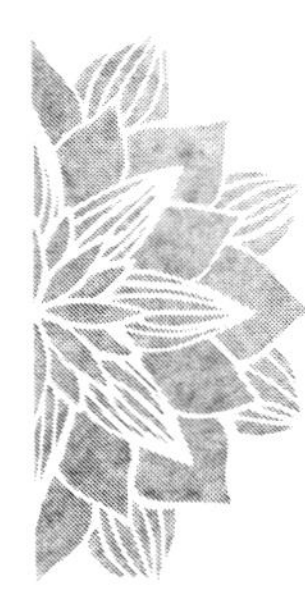

Yoga is the practice of quieting the mind.

Patanjali

9

A Well-Balanced Diet

A suitable diet can restore health at any age.

— *Ayurveda*[1]

Just as over-eating makes the body fat and heavy, so under-eating makes it weak and nervous. The proper balance must therefore be found between the needs of the body and the quantity of food absorbed.

— *Ayurveda*

A well-balanced diet contains a sufficient supply of protein, carbohydrates, fats, salts and minerals. The quantity of food absorbed should correspond to the needs of the body. Both the quantity and the quality of nourishment which the body cells get from the food we eat are important for good health.

1 The Ayurveda is part of one of the four Vedas, the *Atharva-Veda*. The Vedas are the ancient Holy Scriptures of the Hindus, containing the supremo knowledge and highest philosophy. The Ayurveda deals with the Science of Life. It contains all the secrets for keeping the human body in perfect health. This Veda is a treatise in which ways of remedying illness by the use of herbs and plants are to be found. Five or six thousand years ago, the initiated in India already knew that illness was caused by a multitude of minute, invisible creatures, today called 'germs'.

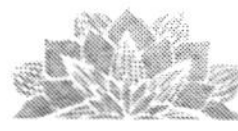

Medical science confirms that the excessive number of calories absorbed in over-eating accumulate in the form of fat and thus accelerate the deterioration of the human body.

What we eat should be fresh, clean and, where possible, untreated. Greasy, fried food should be avoided, for they are bad for the liver. The diet adopted should include increasing amounts of raw foodstuffs, e.g., green salads, vegetables, fruit, cereals, milk and dairy products (cheese and curds), honey. In cold regions, a certain amount of meat and fish may be consumed. Fresh fruit and vegetable juices are also excellent for health.

The three important factors required for a well-balanced diet are:

First, choose nourishing food — energy and vitality can be increased and maintained only through the judicious use of foodstuffs.

Second, eat in moderation, i.e., slightly less than one's fill, because in this way the body feels light, active and energetic. Eating more than we need deforms the body, damages the health, reduces efficiency, and shortens life.

Third, food should be thoroughly masticated (chewed) and mixed with saliva to aid digestion and assimilation. Each mouthful should be chewed ten to fifteen times until it is thoroughly soaked in saliva, reduced to a pulp and then into juice.

Heavy food should be avoided in the evening meal and especially before going to bed.

One should make it a habit never to eat without being hungry, never to fall back on stimulants to prolong the pleasure of eating and satisfy one's greed (what is called a 'civilized' appetite). One should constantly bear in mind that any overloading of the digestive system can lead to numerous illnesses, and that people often 'dig their grave with fork.'

A well-balanced diet is a remarkable asset in maintaining the mind in a perfect state or health and equilibrium, within a body of uniform proportions and perfect fitness.

WATER, A GREAT GIFT OF NATURE FOR MAN'S LIFE AND HEALTH

Drinking plenty of water is important for good health. When thirsty, we should drink water; but slowly, in small sips, and above all avoid gulping it down in one draught. A certain amount of water is essential to stimulate the circulatory system, favour nutrition, help digestion and eliminate the body's waste products. It is required also for the proper functioning of the kidneys, for it forms part of the various juices in the organism, e g., bile, gastric juices, etc.

We should not drink while eating, because such liquids dissolve the gastric juices and pointlessly swells the stomach. Water should be taken half an hour before and after a meal; this is normally suitable for any temperament or condition.

According to the Ayurveda, a glass of water at bedtime and on getting up in the morning will completely wash the organism.

It has been observed that those who do not drink enough water are often anaemic. Their skin dries out and perspiration diminishes. They are nearly always constipated. One should drink at least one litre water a day, and even more if one lives in a hot country.

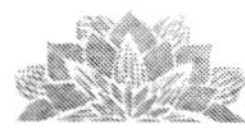

PROTEIN

Protein is responsible for building up a substantial part of the human body and replenish deficiencies caused by illness. One should take care to consume the exact quantity of protein, since excessive intake can prove dangerous to a healthy equilibrium. Soya beans, peanuts, chickpeas, lentils, cheese, milk protein (casein), powdered milk — all of these are rich in protein. Vegetables, milk and fruits also contain protein but in lesser quantity.

FATS

Fats are essential for the conservation of body temperature. They provide us with energy, keep the tendons supple and help us recover lost energy. Without a fair amount of fat, we quickly fall victim to a number of illnesses including: colds, coughs, pneumonia, tuberculosis, etc. Olive oil, peanut oil, sunflower oil, etc., fresh or metted butter, contain fats. Walnuts, pistachio nuts, almonds, hazel nuts, soya beans, rice, lentils, flour, powdered milk, cheese, eggs, oily fish, and meat all contain a certain quantity of fats.

CARBOHYDRATES

Once digested, carbohydrates preserve the body temperature and provide energy. They help digestion, but if eaten in too large a quantity, they cannot be assimilated fully by the body and therefore have an adverse effect on our health and active life.

Foods with a high carbohydrate content are:

(1) Honey, sugar cane, sugar beet, grapes, molasses.

(2) All foods containing starch, such as rice flour, chick peas, peas, lentils, tamarind, turmeric, maize, etc.

(B) Foods with a high carbohydrate content: beetroot, potatoes, onions, carrots, radishes, coconuts, peanuts and other oil-producing nuts, fruits such as the mango, fig, date, banana, and spices such as cardamom, cumin, coriander, ginger, and cloves.

(C) Foods containing less carbohydrate, i.e., the kinds of vegetable, fruit and herbs (except those listed above).

CLASSIFICATION OF FOODSTUFFS ACCORDING TO YOGA AND AYURVEDA

The ancient Rishis of India discovered a simple dietetic treatment that was highly effective against most illnesses, and at the same time lay down certain fundamental principles of good health for general guidance. According to the Sages, there are two main causes for physical illness: over-eating and under-eating. Millions and millions of people are victims of a badly adjusted diet, and the ideal way to correct it is to eat plenty of seasonal vegetables and fruit.

It is known that people follow three types of diet: carnivorous, lacto-vegetarian, and mixed. The majority of population follows mixed diet, i.e., a mixture of vegetables, fruits, cereals, milk and meat.

Those who practise Yoga, especially if they are following the spiritual path, generally adopt the lacto-vegetarian diet, consisting strictly of fruits, vegetables, cereals, nuts, milk and dairy products, honey, and unrefined sugar. This diet allows perfect equilibrium between the processes of assimilation and evacuation, for the natural health of the body, plus the powers of concentration and meditation, depend to a large extent on such functions.

FOODSTUFFS RECOMMENED FOR DAILY DIET

Curd (Yoghurt)

In India, curd is a part of every meal. It is a source of nourishment,

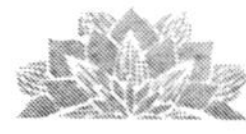

maintaining vigour and virility to a very old age. It also prolongs life. Curd has many advantages; it helps digestion of protein easily and calcium more readily. The B group vitamins produced by curd bacteria in the intestines are of great use. The feeling of heaviness and the excessive gas suffered by many are gradually eliminated.

HONEY

Bees are the greatest manufacturers of sweetmeats. They have far greater skill and produce far healthier sweets than any confectioner, with all his dexterity, ingenuity, and many ingedients, can ever hope to make.

According to Ayurveda, honey is a natural, living food-stuff. It consists of the quintessence of flowers collected by bees, and has wonderful properties for revitalizing the human body. It is one of the most nourishing things one can eat and is also a great tonic, being easy to digest and assimilate. It should be an important part in the nourishment of pregnant women because it regenerates milk. At birth, the baby should have his tongue coated with honey, his first food.

Honey is an incomparable source of energy, fortifying muscles and calming the nerves. It helps one to sleep, and tones up a weak heart, delicate stomach, and flagging brain. Honey regulates the bowel movements efficiently and acts as an agent to restore the calcium content to the bones. It kills germs and helps the body overcome illness; it has also been discovered that germs carrying disease cannot grow in honey. It can be used as a substitute for orange juice and cod liver oil, and is helpful, due to its antiseptic properties, in combating colds, flu, sore throat, coughs, bronchial catarrh, stomachache, and throat infections.

Honey is an effective remedy for anaemia and constipation. Circulation is improved by it and so is the functioning of the liver.

It contains many vitamins and organic acids, which help in the assimilation of food and protect against illness. If one is tired, over-worked or depressed, a teaspoon of honey in hot water acts as an instant pick-me-up. Honey and soaked almonds may be used against mental sluggishness, for it is a powerful tonic for the brain. A dozen almonds are soaked overnight in warm water, and their skin removed in the morning. The almonds are eaten with two teaspoons of honey. Within a few days, one will feel full of energy and life.

A teaspoon of honey a day will keep the stomach and bowels in good condition for the rest of our lives.

In India, those who practise Ayurvedic medicine, give a daily dose of juice of two or three well ripened lemons, the grated peel and mixed with honey to patients of rheumatism. It is indeed a good idea to eat one lemon a day; its juice mixed with a teaspoon of honey prevents acidity.

N.B. People often ask if honey is fattening. In fact, the opposite is true, Honey is recommended during a slimming diet because it is very quickly absorbed, unlike other sugars which are 'metabolized' more slowly, causing fat to accumulate. This is why honey, when taken in small quantities, is not only a wonderful health food, but enables one to stay slim.

WHEAT GERM

Wheat germ constitutes the essential part from which the wheat plant sprouts. It is one of the richest sources of vitamins B_1, B_2, B_{12}, PP[2] and E; proteins, fats and iron are also present in it. Specialists of Ayurveda recommend wheat germ and its oil to be included in our daily meals. The oil or germ may be mixed in salads, cereals and soups, or eaten with cottage cheese, curd or fresh fruit salad or

2 PP is also known as Vitamin B3/Niacin/Nicotinic acid

sprink it on bread and butter, or put it in sandwiches. Wheat germ is exceptionally energy-giving.

How to make homemade wheat germ

Wash a handful of wheat and put it in a bowl of warm water. Soak for at least twenty-four hours, then rinse in warm water. Put it onto an earthenware plate which will preserve constant humidity: the wheat will sprout very quickly.

SOYA

Soya is a complete food that is easy to digest and provides energy. It is particularly recommended to those who are tired, nervous or anaemic, because the substances composing soya powerfully regenerate the muscles, liver and bones.

Soya may be eaten in the form of beans, seeds, oil or flour. Those who are unable to drink animal milk may use soya milk as a substitute.

Soya proteins incorporate all the amino-acids required by the organism, thus making it one of the most balanced food.

POWDERED MILK

Powdered milk is very common nowadays, especially for prescribed diets. It is without doubt a highly nourishing drink, which, if mixed with fresh milk, is rich in protein, calcium and other vitamins, especially vitamin B_2 and contains hardly any fat. Nevertheless, the Ayurveda specialists do not consider that it should be substituted for fresh milk.

During the process of drying, dehydrated milk loses its vital contents and natural properties; it becomes a concentrate and product of milk, like any other derivative product. Fresh milk is more easily digested and assimilated into the system, and it nourishes the whole body.

MOLASSES

Molasses in India is called 'Rab'. It is an unrefined product of sugar cane, very rich in iron, calcium, vitamin B and all other minerals. It tastes very good and can be mixed with milk, fruit juice, curd and may even be used as a substitute for sugar. Molasses also possess excellent laxative qualities. It invigorates the muscles and stimulates the whole nervous system.

DATES

The Sanskrit word for dates is 'Kharjur'; there are fresh dates and dried ones. They are good, rejuvenating food, and are rich in substances for regenerating the body. Dates tone up the body, but are fattening when eaten in too great a quantity. They contain 70% of body-nourishing elements that are easily absorbed, such as fructose, calcium, iron, magnesium, potassium, phosphorus, alkalies, and vitamins A, D, B_1, C in normal proportions. In addition, dates increase the quantity of seminal fluid and add to sexual potency. To regain the latter the following tonic drink should be taken:

Soak two or three dried dates overnight in an earthenware bowl filled with water. By the next morning they will have swelled, and one can remove the stones and boil the date flesh in half a litre of fresh milk. Basic sexual energy will be regained by eating the dates and drinking the milk which also acts as a tonic.

Dates possess other well-known properties, e.g., to rid oneself of a burning sensation inside the body, two or three dates should be mashed in 250 ml of water, which is then filtered through a piece of cloth and drunk. The effect may be accelerated by using rose water instead of ordinary water.

Dates are very nourishing, therefore, energy-giving and a good tonic for nerves and muscles. They also prevent senility and even cancer.

Gandhiji ate dates as part of his diet for a very long time. Dates and milk make a very healthy breakfast, especially in winter.

FIGS

Figs are an ideal nutritive food and take a prominent place among fruit. They are extremely good for the health and are easily digested. They regulate the liver and spleen functions, and remove constipation. Dried or fresh figs may be included in daily diet. They contain vitamins A, B_1, B_2, PP, C, several proteins, carbohydrates, sugar, iron, sodium, sulphur, magnesium, calcium and bromine.

Figs are highly nutritious and digestible restoratives; they should be eaten, not only by sportsmen, but also by children, adolescents, convalescents, old people, and especially pregnant women. As figs are very rich in necessary nutritional substances, they enable one to recuperate quickly after physical and mental effort, and ensure the body vitality and renewed force. It is strongly recommended, therefore, to include figs in one's daily diet.

TOMATOES

Tomatoes are a very important vegetable; they have a savory taste, and their acidity is not pungent. They contain vitamins A, B, (B_1, B_2, B_3) C, D, PP, E, K, and are rich in sulphur, potassium, iron, calcium and magnesium. Tomatoes also contain copper, zinc and iodine.

The vitamins contained in tomatoes are not destroyed when cooked but they lose a certain number of vitamins on boiling.

Tomatoes are best eaten raw. They stimulate the nervous system and purify blood. Constipation is cured and the teeth strengthened. Tomatoes are easily digested, which is why they are recommended for invalids, especially diabetics and those who are feverish.

Experience has shown that tomatoes regulate the amount of sugar in the urine of diabetics. Being rich in vitamin A, they are very useful as a preventive measure against nocturnal blindness, short-sightedness, and other eye problems.

Being a rich source of vitamins and mineral salts, especially vitamin C, calcium and iron, tomatoes are very beneficial for the health of growing children; one teaspoon of fresh tomato juice three times a day is sufficient for a one year-old child.

CARROTS

Carrots are considered an extraordinarily useful vegetable if one wants to follow a balanced diet. They are very good for the development and growth of the body. They also help strengthen immunity against various illnesses.

In India, there are two types of carrot: one dark red and the other orange. Both are unusually rich in vitamin A. They also contain vitamins B and C, plus carotene (provitamin A), iron, phosphorus, sulphur, calcium, sodium, potassium, and magnesium are present as well. Sugar, dextrose and levulose are also to be found in them; these substances get assimilated directly. Carrots also contain-a few proteins. It has been observed that the iron contained in carrots may be more directly assimilated than that from medical supplements.

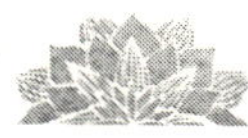

If eaten regularly, carrots afford effective protection against contagious diseases, such as sinusitis, or other eye and ear disorders. They also relieve burning sensations when urinating. Hyperacidity may be treated by drinking carrot juice in the morning and evening.

Carrots are a good remedy against gastric or stomach ulcers, and chronic constipation. Liver complaints, bilious disorders, jaundice and urinary problems are cured by eating cooked carrots or drinking fresh carrot juice in a substantial quantity.

It has been proved that certain skin diseases may be cured and the complexion and physical beauty enhanced by eating carrots for fifteen to twenty days. Carrot juice is particularly effective against scabies, anaemia, *scrofula* and impurities of the blood. To gain the maximum advantage, one should eat carrots raw or take fresh carrot juice. It tones up the body, removes toxins, provides the organism with minerals, re-establishes its balance, and fortifies the tissues and cells.

N.B. It is better to scrape or brush the carrots in cold water rather than peel them: the skin is very rich in vitamins.

Being rich in vitamin A, carrots can replace milk, olive oil and cod liver oil. They are particularly suitable for those who do not like milk or cod liver oil.

GINGER

Ginger is a spicy root used in cooking, as a syrup, and for medical purposes. It may be used fresh or in powdered form. It is very good for maintaining body heat and regulating body temperature. Ginger contains vitamin C and Flavonoids, as well as iodine, iron, potassium and sulphur. It helps relieve rheumatism and arthritis, soothes bodily pains, and is effective in combating bad chills. It may be included in soup or used to add flavour to cooked vegetables.

Ginger helps in digestion and elimination of wind. Ginger may also be used in cakes, biscuits, etc.

Care should be taken in using ginger by persons sensitive to spicy flavour. This is how it can be used to maximum advantage: take a fresh ginger root and grate a very small quantity (half a teaspoon). Mix into soup or cooked vegetables just before serving, simply to add flavour.

Ginger may also be used as a tea; a teaspoon of pure honey and a few drops of lemon should be added to taste.

LEMON

Lemons are rich in vitamin C, which is required to ensure normal digestion. If absent from daily diet, gastric and sanguinary troubles my ensue. Lemons have high vitamin A content, very important for growth, considerable quantities of B_1, B_2, B_3, indispensable for the balance of the nervous system, and vitamin B_3 or niacin, which protects the vascular system. Lemons also contain iron, calcium, silica, phosphorus, magnesium and copper.

Lemon helps eliminate wind and bile, and stimulates the digestive system. It protects against intestinal worms, stomachaches, and loss of appetite. Lemon is also useful in relieving digestive troubles, disorders of the nervous system, and in re-establishing the equilibrium of the fundamental elements of the body.

It is recommended to drink the fresh juice of half a lemon in the evening to fight off dyspepsia (indigestion), vomiting and headaches induced by the malfunctioning of the liver.

Six to fifteen grams of lemon juice mixed with twenty grams of water, morning and evening after meals, constitutes an excellent remedy for liver complaints, constipation, stomachache, loss of appetite (anorexia), and wind.

A little lemon juice, taken every six hours, will calm nervous pains and reduce arterial tension. Lemon reduces abnormally high temperatures during intermittent attacks of malaria.

The raging thirst and high temperatures that accompany fever may be relieved by taking lemon syrup, i.e., 15 to 20 grams of lemon juice in hot water. It is a very effective remedy against cholera. The bad effects of narcotics, opium or alcohol will be dispersed by the consumption of lemon juice. It also helps relieve vomiting and eliminates flatulence.

The daily use of lemon and sea-salt is an excellent remedy against dilation of the spleen. Lemon syrup relieves unsual sensation of heat or burning, heart palpitations, constipation and retention of urine.

One part of lemon mixed together with two parts of glycerine applied to the face, hands and feet at bedtime will soften the skin.

One part of lemon mixed together with two parts of olive oil, applied all over the body and rubbed in, will soften skin and give it lustre, removing the dryness and dirt from the body.

Soup or vegetables seasoned with lemon make it more appetizing and easier to digest.

Lemon juice with salt, black pepper, cominoes and coriander stimulates appetite, regulates bowel movements, and relieves wind and flatulence.

Salt water and lemon juice is a common remedy in India against over-eating or rich food. In India, practitioners of Ayurveda give patients of rheumatism, sciatica, lumbago, or pains in the hip joints, a daily dose of the juice of two or three ripe lemons mixed with grated skin and honey. It is a good idea to eat at least one lemon a day. Lemon juice does not hurt if mixed with a teaspoon of honey; it prevents hyper-acidity.

ONIONS

Onions are so commonly used in kitchens of almost every home. Onion juice is an aphrodisiac, stimulant and expectorant. Onions contain a large quantity of vitamins A, B, C, iron, iodine, sulphur, sodium, potassium, nitrates and phosphates of calcium, silicon, etc. Sugars and soluble carbohydrates are also to be found in onions.

Although raw onions lend an unpleasant odour to the breath, raw onions, rather than fried or cooked, are best for disinfecting the alimentary canal. When eaten raw, onion also has a diuretic effect.

There are two kinds of onions, one white, the other red. They are piquant in flavour, but are very nourishing and help to calm coughs. They stimulate the appetite, act as a tonic and, although slightly less easily digested, constitute excellent antidotes. They also soothe stomachache, relieve flatulence and increase semen.

The red, alkaline onion has a bitter taste, sometimes sweet, which stimulates the appetite. It is extremely soporific, but calms a dry throat. Bile and toxins in the body disappear with this onion.

Onion seeds cure dental infections and urinary diseases. Onions should be regularly included in diet; they protect the roots of the teeth from all sorts of infection and prevent dental problems.

Many kinds of migraine may be treated by the application of onion pulp to the soles of the feet.

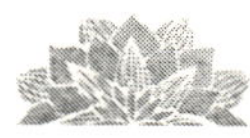

In the case of fainting, the patient should be made to inhale a few drops of onion juice at short invervals; this helps to regain consciousness quickly.

Onions prepared in vinegar soothe stomachache, are an excellent digestive and appetizer, and have been tested against numerouss diseases of the spleen, where they have been shown to reduce dilation to a normal level. They are also a remedy against anaemia. To prepare them, chop the onions into small pieces, add pure vineger, salt, black pepper and cumin.

Onion juice mixed with mustard oil is a good remedy to massage into inflamed joints; it reduces the inflammation and allows the joints to move normally.

GARLIC

Garlic has been known since ancient times. It is added to food in every country. It has a very strong odour and pungent flavour. To take away the smell of garlic one should chew a few grains of aniseed, coffee beans, cardamom seeds, fennel, cumin, or simply suck a slice of lemon. Garlic is an effective antiseptic. Its essence is often used for various medical preparations.

Garlic contains sulphur, iodine, silicon, starch, sulphurized glucoside, allium oxide, etc. It stimulates and re-establishes the equilibrium of the glands, serves as an intestinal and pulmonary antiseptic, dissolves uric acid, and renders the blood more fluid. Garlic is a diuretic substance, a vasodilator and hypotenser against gout, and an agent against sclerosis, arthritis, rheumatism, and asthma. A few drops of garlic on a piece of sugar will help calm an attack of asthma. Garlic activates the digestion and eliminates flatulence. It is an excellent remedy against high blood pressure, cardiac fatigue, vascular spasms, circulatory troubles, varicose veins, haemorroids, and glandular imbalances.

Garlic in cooked food is good for general health, and should be added raw to salads.

Two cloves of chopped garlic together with a few sprigs of parsley and a few drops of olive oil may be applied on bread and eaten, for breakfast.

A good remedy for rheumatism is to take one part of garlic and two parts of camphor oil and massage it into the body. Rubbing it along the spinal column helps to eliminate general weakness and debility. Wasp and insect stings can be soothed immediately by rubbing garlic on them.

According to Ayurveda, garlic cloves placed in a small bag worn around the neck of a patient or applied to the navel provide protection against worms and many infectious diseases.

AN IDEAL DIET

According to both Ayurveda and Yoga, food is responsible for the individual's physical, mental and spiritual development. Since food is the source of vitality, errors in diet will lead to disorders. This is why we should be well aware of the properties of the food we eat.

In India, Ayurveda and Yoga categorise food into three: *satvik* (pure or superior quality), *rajasik* (medium quality) and *tamasik* (inferior quality).

Satvik foods help maintain the body's health, give it strength and vitality, render it immune to illness, and create physical, mental and spiritual balance. *Satvik* therefore means ideal or superior quality food. Such foods are easy-to-digest and does not cause uric acid or other toxins to accumulate in the body. By consuming *satvik* foods or following a diet of ideal food, one may preserve one's strength to old age without illness. This is why *satvik* preserves the body and mind in peace and perfect equilibrium.

In *satvik* category, are included fruits, vegetables, green salads, lentils, milk, curd, cottage cheese, fresh butter, hazelnuts, almonds, dried fruit, honey, rice and food with small quantities of whole wheat flour.

Nowadays, it is thought that a well-balanced ideal diet in the *rajasik* category (medium quality) may include vegetarian and partly non-vegetarian foods, i.e., *satvik* food with concentrated combined products such as melted butter, sugar, sweets, fried foods, meat, fish, eggs, etc. Unfortunately, both these varieties of food are cooked in oil and other greasy substances. They are fried, over-spiced, accompanied with sauces that enrich the flavour but destory the *satvik* (pure) element and other food values, thus causing illness and pain.

N.B. Boiling food, e.g., meat, fish, cabbage, spinach, etc., destroys the necessary vital elements in them. Steaming is therefore recommended, with the use of the natural humidity of the foodstuffs and the smallest amount of heat possible.

Yoga allows adolescents and adults up to the age of forty-five to consume *rajasik* food (medium quality) in moderation. It strongly advises against *rajasik* for those who are over fifty or have chosen the spiritual path and can only eat *satvik* foods.

In the *tamasik* (inferior quality) category, we find food which is stale, unclean, rotten, decomposed or dried up. It has an adverse effect on physical and mental balance.

It is known that all the organs of the body receive nourishment and vitality through the bloodstream. According to Ayurveda, food may be divided into two groups: alkaline and acid. One group produces predominantly alkaline blood, and the other predominantly acid.

The function of acid blood is to provide the body with energy and to make good its deficiencies. Alkaline blood nourishes the organs, such as the nerves, glands, bones, marrow, etc. It is also the force motivating these organs; it maintains the human machine in working order, both physically and mentally. It destroys germs and protects the body from illness.

In the alkaline category, i.e., alkaline blood producing after digestion, we find sweet and sour fruit, green vegetables, various kinds of lentils, milk, curd, butter and honey, etc. All the mineral salts and vitamins of the alkaline category are also to be found in them.

The liver and pancreas are glands of the digestive system. When overloaded with rich or highly concentrated foods, they weaken and hence function poorly, leading to illness. Extreme caution is therefore required, both by healthy and sick people, when dealing with this category of foodstuffs. A well-balanced, ideal diet is needed to preserve the body in good health.

If people knew how to eat properly, they would develop both spiritually and mentally, would remain healthy and vigorous, and live at least for one hundred years.

HOW TO OVERCOME PREMATURE OLD AGE

Generally speaking, the idea of growing old gives rise to much apprehension. Nobody wants to 'get on in years'. The known controllable causes of premature ageing are worry, nervous tension, inadequate rest, lack of adequate exercise and wrong diet.

Many people abuse their body, lead an irregular life far removed from nature, and thus wear out before they have had a chance to discover the elixir of youth. How can those who use drugs, artificial stimulants and tranquillizers hope to be in good health? It is regrettable that the majority are completely unaware of this state of affairs.

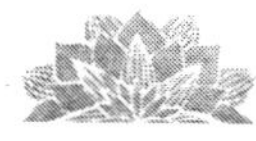

Science has discovered the reason for ageing: it is not a sickness, but a combination of factors. One of them is the absence of hormone secretions, which affect the ageing process and hasten death.

According to certain schools of medicine, the human body completely renews itself every seven years, i.e., it is reconstituted by the constant replacement of old cells by new ones. The rate at which these are created depends on the level of our vibrations and on whether our thoughts are optimistic or depressing. We do indeed transform the body — ourselves at every instant of our life, improving it or making it deteriorate according to our thoughts.

It has been discovered that both men and women can change their looks by the power of thought and the regular practice of Yoga under supervision. Such people may look and be exactly as they wish as a result of their own efforts. Those already marked by age may regain their youth and thus prolong their lives.

Examination of the various causes of ageing show that it is a slow and progressive process, in the course of which the different parts of the body lose their elasticity. As the percentage of mineral substances grows, so the bones become more brittle, and the signs of age begin to set in.

The body's elasticity also depends on the state of the blood vessels. Gradual accumulation of sedimentary deposits such as lime, chalk, etc., in the arterial and venous walls, causes loss of elasticity in these blood vessels. There can be no doubt that as we advance in years, so these deposits engender arterial sclerosis, i.e., the blocking of arteries by chalky deposits, resulting in a general deterioration of the physical state. Such impurities may be traced back to defective breathing, insufficient or improper exercise, harmful indulgence, an artificial way of life and wrong diet. The faster the deposits accumulate, the faster one grows old.

The elasticity of the muscles plays an important part in the preservation of the body's youth. We may lose this elasticity by accumulating an abnormally large quantity of fats, spread evenly or unevenly throughout the body. Such fats may be caused by an inactive life. Bad digestion is also the cause of abnormal fat deposits; it can harden the muscular tissue. An abnormal volume of fat prevents the tissues from fulfilling their role and completely assimilating the required amounts of nutritional substances from the bloodstream. It also hinders the movements of the muscles and impedes the vital parts of the body, e.g., the heart, lungs, stomach, bowels, from fulfilling their respective functions in suitable conditions.

Even athletes are not immune from the adverse effects of abnormal accumulations of fat. By the practise Yoga system, however, we can preserve the elasticity of youth, eliminate the growth of mineral deposits in the bones, check and prevent the accumulation of sedimentary deposits, and, if there is already an excessive quantity in the blood vessels, reduce the surplus fat to a minimum. Thus we may, to a large extent, regain our lost youth.

What actually happens during the process of ageing? Between the ages of 30 and 90, the weight of the muscles decreases by 30%, and likewise our strength. The number of fibres that compose a nerve is reduced by one quarter. The weight of the brain is noticeably diminished, for dead cells are not replaced, and all the physical functions are slowed down. The muscles lose their strength, the heart pumps less blood and takes longer to recuperate after physical effort: at the age of ninety, the volume of blood being pumped is only half that of age twenty. The lungs filter less air, so have to work harder to obtain a given quantity of oxygen. Why is this?

In recent years, it has been noted with almost complete certainty that this is due to the accidental failure and possible death of individual cells in the body, each dying off one after another. Death is often caused by cardiac arrest because the heart is a muscle whose cells are not replaced when they die. If one of the vital organs is subjected to violent effort, or weakened by infection, it will be the first to 'give up'. Hence a remedy to prevent cells from dying would preserve the strength of youth and prolong our lives. Let us examine the case of muscular strength: A man aged 70 usually only has the same strength as he had at the age of 12 or 13 — roughly half that of 20. Muscular strength depends on the volume of protein, but the human body's capacity to produce protein depends on the existence of the male hormone testosterone.

It has recently been discovered that the physical factor may be controlled by our psyche one. The psyche often has an influence over the secretion of hormones, which is indeed controlled by the emotions.

As far as prolonging life is concerned, hibernation plays an important part. It allows us to reach a great 'chronological' age, but the time gained in this way escapes the control of the consciousness. Recently, there has been much talk of 'freezing' the body and thus preserving it for a certain time. Hibernation is different from sleep: the body temperature falls, in some cases below zero degrees. The heart beats no more than three times a minute and breathing can be reduced to one breath every three minutes. This 'unconscious hibernation' could therefore last for the whole of life, but the evacuation and adaptation mechanisms would also be slowed down, so that we might not feel particularly well-rested on waking.

It has been discovered that the state of super-consciousness (Samadhi) — the ultimate goal of the spiritual life — provides the best possible conditions for hibernation. In a state of super-consciousness, the cardiac and respiratory rhythms are reduced to a minimum, so that the energy spent in maintaining life is much less.

Hibernation is nevertheless a state which does not provide the individual with lucidity, whereas in the state of super-consciousness, lucidity is at its maximum.

Important discoveries in the field of deep sleep made in the recent past show that the state of deep sleep is an active one. Until now, it was thought that it was passive; today science has revolutionized this concept. The extraordinary thing is that Hindu Sages arrived at the same conclusion intuitively two thousand years ago. In the *Mandukya Upanishad*, there is a verse which says that sleep is the most regenerative state, because in sleep we identify ourselves with the universal consciousness.

The Yogis attach great importance to the spinal column and its junction with the brain. They tell us that the Sushumna, or hollow channel inside the spinal column, is the passage of very elevated spiritual and mystical experiences (see the chapter on the Nadis, Chakras and Kundalini). The vital importance of the spinal column is clearly shown in several inverted Yogic postures, such as Viparitakarani, Sarvangasana and Sirshasana, which abundantly irrigate the juncture. They also allow this region to be regenerated and help relax it.

We should now turn our attention to the effectiveness of rhythmic and alternate breathing, a remedy suggested by Yoga against the ageing of muscles. Firstly, rhythmic breathing makes it easier to absorb more oxygen, let us remember that oxygen helps transform food into protein and calcium. It is the muscle's inability to assimilate protein that makes it old. Next, rhythmic breathing helps us establish equilibrium between the basis of the nervous and neuro-vegetative systems. The demands of modern life make us spend far more nervous energy than we gain, and it is only in finding a balance between what we spend and what we gain that we are able to maintain our capacity for good health.

There is nothing surprising about Yogis who are able to live by eating hardly anything; the amount of energy they spend is reduced to a minimum and with the remaining energy they are able to establish between the two bases. I have myself seen, with my

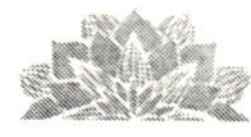

own eyes, a 90-year old Yogi who looked no older than 40-45. Not everybody can, of course, be a real Yogi, but it is certain that if the ageing process can be accelerated, it is reasonable to suppose that it may also be retarded — even stopped — by the regular practice of Yoga, which also allows the individual to become younger.

The three sorts of movement in breathing — to the centre, to the sides and upwards — are effective for all the self-regulated and self-regulating functions, such as the sympathetic and glandular systems, and the flow of blood to the brain. Yoga also declares that rhythmic breathing can change anxiety by acting on the sympathetic nerve and the thalamus.

Yoga therefore teaches us that the body may be put into perfect order and brought under the strict control of the mind. Age is no obstacle, nobody is too old to start Yoga. Those who are physically unable to perform difficult postures can nevertheless carry out the appropriate breathing, relaxation, and a few simplified postures, designed to render the joints more supple by lubricating them in such a way that the circulation and vital energy remain in perfect condition.

CONCLUSION

Yoga provides us with three weapons against premature old age.

First, is to invert the body so that the volume of arterial blood reaching the head is increased, thus irrigating the brain, stimulating mental vigour, nourishing the skin and facial tissues, preventing and softening wrinkles.

The second is Pranayama (controlled rhythmic and alternate breathing); a tired body may be completely recharged with energy by Pranayama, just as a battery may be recharged by connecting it to the current.

The third weapon is a well-balanced diet. I have already observed that those who practise Yoga under my guidance have become younger in body and face, have increased their vitality and improved their intellectual abilities. Virility in men and menstruation in ageing women will be renewed at a large extent. This method helps us to remain young and full of vitality, thus prolonging life.

HOW TO LEAD A WELL-BALANCED AND CONTROLLED SEX LIFE

I have often been asked if there are any standard rules or guidelines concerning normal sex life. The need for sexual liberation is a matter of individual discretion, and it is impossible to define what is 'normal' or 'average' sexual activity. Nevertheless, one cannot deny that a balanced and controlled sex life is important. Everybody reacts differently according to his own temperament. One thing is certain, however, and that is that each individual has the capacity to control his sex life and regulate it according to his own desires.

Many people have very little understanding of what love is. They think that love springs solely from the desire for sexual union, to satisfy mutual desires. Freud and various other psychiatrists tell us that the sexual instinct results from a chemically produced tension of which the body must rid itself.

Sexual instinct is indeed a natural human desire. It is paternal for man and maternal for woman, and leads them firstly to reproduce, without which the human race would not continue, and secondly to enjoy physical sensations, which have a biological basis.

The practice of Yoga does not present any obstacle to marriage. A large number of Yogis and Sages of ancient India, along with medieval mystics from various civilizations, led a totally normal married life, which did not stop them from achieving their aims.

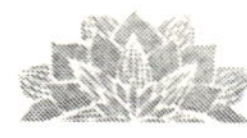

All Yogic texts agree that the suppression of sexual desire and forced continence are irrational. Medical science and psychiatry have also shown that forced abstinence can lead to frustration and perversion, which are the causes of neurotic tendencies. Sexual desire should be sublimated and transformed, not suppressed, for suppression can do much harm and become the source of constant agitation.

Yoga is not intended exclusively for celibates. Continence is a state of mind, whether one is married or not. It is not a negation, imposed austerity or prohibition, but a way of disciplining and controlling our thoughts. For sensuality does not only reside in the body or senses, it is also in our thoughts; we therefore have to learn to control and discipline our thoughts as well.

The great Yogis of India have perfected a discipline and offer it to humanity. They teach us how to balance our sexual energy, to regulate and control it through breathing, regular practice of the Asanas, the Mudras (endurance postures), and Bandhas (postures in which certain organs of the body are contracted and controlled), so that anyone, whatever their individual needs, may follow their teachings without difficulty. Thus they may draw great therapeutic benefit from them and lead a happy, well-balanced and self-controlled life.

The Yoga discipline is applicable to all:
— the married, who lead both a family and social life.
— those with neurotic, psychological and psychic problems.
— those who have renounced the world to follow the spiritual path and lead a life of complete chastity so that they may divert their sexual energy to higher nervous centres, thus to attain the Goal more quickly, i e., Self-realization.

10

Useful Hints

As the wind gathers the clouds then scatters them, so the mind creates ties and breaks them.

— *Shankaracharya*

REST AND RELAXATION

We may easily learn to relax and rest by practising Savasana and rhythmic breathing. This will improve our sleep and regularly recharge the body with vital energy. Through Yogic relaxation, the mind becomes calm and is like a radio transmitter emitting waves of inner tranquility and vibrations of peace. It is only then that we experience true rest.

SLEEP

It is very important to go to bed at ten in the evening, ten thirty at the latest. This is because before midnight the cosmic position of the earth provides the most favourable radiation for the regeneration of our nervous system. It is said that the best hours for sleep and complete rest are ten in the evening and four in the morning.

TOBACCO, DRUGS AND ALCOHOL

It is better to abstain from smoking and avoid alcoholic beverages. Tobacco and alcohol destory the nervous centres that Yoga seeks to animate. Abuse of them leads not only to a deterioration of health, but also of mental force and vigour.

Drugs should be avoided at all costs. They harm the nervous and digestive system, and ruin the freshness of the complexion. They are a veritable poison for the body and mind. They reduce the mental faculties, and destroy the will-power and resistance.

BATHS

One should take a bath or shower every day, but never immediately after performing Asanas or Pranayama exercises; it is best to wait at least half an hour. Nor should one take a bath after meals before the food has been properly digested. In cases where it is difficult to take a bath or take a bath or shower every day, these may be replaced by a thorough wash-down. This gives the skin a chance to breathe, since it is continually covered in a thick layer of clothes and does not therefore receive enough air.

AIRINGS OR 'AIRBATHING'

This means that once every so often one removes the clothing, allowing the pores to breathe freely. This is extremely good for the body and improves the exterior tone of the neurovegetative system so that the body develops a wonderful power of resistance.

SUNBATHING

Another form of bathing is sunbathing. It is a source of energy and force, provided it is practised carefully and deliberately. The sun's rays are a marvellous tonic, but they should not be abused.

We should sit in the shade beside a river, lake or the sea, and allow the sun's rays to reflect off the water on to us In this way they are even more beneficial than direct rays. If the sun is hidden by clouds or mist, the effect of its filtered rays is very powerful and one tans just as easily. The best time for sunbathing is the morning, at dawn when the sun has just risen. This is the time when it can cure many illnesses. It provides us with vitamin D and gives us warmth and vitality.

SWIMMING

If we have an opportunity to swim in a river, lake or the sea, especially in summer, we should take as much advantage of it as we can. Particularly by swimming in the sea, the skin is toned up by the minerals, iodine and the pure air, which is extremely rich in ozone. Swimming is the best exercise for regulating and controlling breathing, and this is extremely beneficial to health.

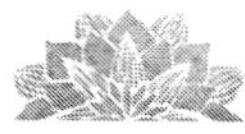

NOSE BATH

Should one have a cold, fill a bowl with water as hot as one can stand and add a teaspoon of biocarbonate of soda or sea-salt, plunge the nose into the bowl inhaling the water through the nostrils until it flows into the throat. Eject through the mouth. Next practice *Viparitakarani* or *Sarvangasana*. By performing this treatment two or three times a day — but never after meals — one may be sure of getting rid of the most stubborn cold.

WALKING BAREFOOT

Whenever we can, and especially in good weather, we should walk barefoot in fields and meadows, beside rivers, lakes and the sea. This is because the soles of the feet absorb the earth's radiation thus fortifying and refreshing the whole organism to an amazing degree.

EATING

Meals should be eaten in moderation. Food should be thoroughly masticated (chewed), so that it is mixed with saliva and may be absorbed and assimilated by the organism more easily. The consumption of meat is permitted in cold countries, but it must be pointed out that this substance introduces many toxins and waste-products if eaten in excess, thus severely taxing the digestive organs.

Yoga experiments affirm that all food, such as raw and green vegetables, fruit and fresh fruit juices, milk and dairy products and honey are filled with Prana (vital force) which is of supreme importance for the maintenance of life, energy and health..

A YOGA LESSON

(of about thirty minutes)

1.	**Complete Yogic Breathing, Lying on back**	5 times
	or Sitting cross-legged	5 times
2.	**Pavana Muktasana**	5 to 7 times
3.	**Bhujangasana**	2 to 3 times, 5 seconds
4.	**Ardha-Salabhasana**	2 times
5.	**Paschimottanasana or Padahastasana**	5 seconds; repeat 2 to 3 times 5 seconds; repeat 3 to 5 times
6.	**Vakrasana**	5 seconds on each side
7.	**Trikonasana**	repeat 2 times
8.	**Viparitakarani**	5 seconds to 1 minute; add 15 sec. per week until 1 min.
9.	**Yoga-Mudra**	2 to 3 times
10.	**Anuloma Viloma**	2 to 5 rounds
11.	**Ujjayi Pranayama**	3 to 7 rounds
12.	**Savasana**	2 minutes; add 2 min. per week until 10 min.

A YOGA LESSON

(of about one hour)

1.	**Complete Yogic Breathing, Lying on back or Sitting cross-legged**	5 times 5 times
2.	**Padmasana or Siddhasana**	5 seconds; add 10 sec. per week until 3 min.
3.	**Bhujangasana**	2 to 3 times; 5 sec.
4.	**Salabhasana**	2 to 3 times; 5 sec.
5.	**Dhanurasana**	2 to 3 times; 5 sec.
6.	**Paschimottonasana**	5 seconds each side; repeat 2 to 3 times
7.	**Halasana**	2 to 60 seconds; repeat 2 to 3 times
8.	**Ardha-Matsyendrasana**	5 seconds; each side repeat 2 to 3 times
9.	**Supta-Vajrasana**	5 seconds; add 5 sec. per week until 1 min.
10.	**Trikonasana**	2 to 3 times
11.	**Sarvangasana**	30 seconds; add 30 sec. per week until 3 min.
12.	**Matsyasana**	5 to 10 breaths as in complete Yogic Breathing
13.	**Sirshasana**	15 seconds; add 15 sec. per week until 3 min.
14.	**Yoga-Mudra**	2 to 3 times from 5 to 10 seconds
15.	**Savasana**	1 to 2 minutes
16.	**Uddiyana-Bandha**	6 times; add 2 times per week until 12 times
17.	**Kapalabhati**	2 to 3 rounds to begin; add 1 round per week depending on ability
18.	**Anuloma Viloma**	2 to 5 times
19.	**Ujjayi Pranayama**	2 to 3 rounds to begin
20.	**Savasana**	2 minutes; add 2 min. per week until 10 min.